Rosacea Diet

Rosacea Diet

◆

A Simple Method to Control Rosacea

Vegetarian and Omnivore Friendly!

Brady Barrows

Writers Club Press
New York Lincoln Shanghai

Rosacea Diet
A Simple Method to Control Rosacea

Writers Club Press
an imprint of iUniverse, Inc.

For information address:
iUniverse, Inc.
2021 Pine Lake Road, Suite 100
Lincoln, NE 68512
www.iuniverse.com

ISBN: 0-595-22800-3

Printed in the United States of America

Legal Disclaimer

The information contained in this book is not meant to substitute for medical care or treatment. Nothing takes the place of speaking with your doctor or other health care professional. You should consult with your doctor or health care provider before changing your current diet. Your rosacea may take longer than thirty days to control using the *Rosacea Diet*. Please consult with your doctor or other health care professional before using any drug product discussed within this book. Rosacea seems to be an individual case by case disease, and the *Rosacea Diet* alone may not control your rosacea and may require additional or other treatment from a qualified physician, including prescription medication, or treatment from a qualified health care practitioner using some other method or treatment. There is no known cure for rosacea, only treatment to control it. There are no implied statements in this book that the *Rosacea Diet* cures rosacea nor is there any claim made in this book or anywhere that the *Rosacea Diet* cures rosacea, but is instead intended only as a way to control rosacea.

www.rosacea-diet.com

To my wife, Betty,
who put up with my hours and hours writing this book.

Contents

Preface

According to the National Rosacea Society[1] rosacea is a chronic, acne-like condition of the facial skin that may affect as many as 14 million Americans, which is 1 in 20. The *Medical Reporter*[2] says that number may be up to 20 Million! The number of rosacea sufferers is growing all over the world. While there is no specific test for rosacea[3], a physician diagnoses it, and may classify it[4]. I am diagnosed with rosacea. Someone who suffers from rosacea is a *rosacean*. In 1999 I experimented with posting some information I discovered about rosacea on my own homepage, then graduated to my first commercial site, mumbet.com, and then to rosacea-control.com, which site is dedicated to

---

1. http://www.rosacea.org
2. http://medicalreporter.health.org/tmr0596/rosacea.html
3. **No Specific Test for Rosacea**
    "…There is no specific test for rosacea, but its characteristic appearance, cutaneous distribution, discrete course, typical target population, and response to various therapies make accurate diagnosis possible.…

    …It is estimated that rosacea occurs in about 13 million (1 in 20) Americans. Onset occurs between 30 and 50 years of age in about half of patients.

    Rosacea appears to occur most often in fair-skinned people of northern and eastern European descent, particularly Celtic, English, and Scottish. It often affects multiple members of the same family, presumably because of their similar complexions and genetic heritage.…"—source of article >
    http://www.postgradmed.com/issues/1999/02_99/millikan.htm
4. **Four Classifications of Rosacea**
    The National Rosacea Society developed a new standard classification system that divides rosacea into four subtypes: **erythematotelangiectatic, papulopustular, phymatous, and ocular.**

    source > http://www.rosacea.org/rr/2002/summer/article_1.html

posting information on the control of rosacea, and to advertise the *Rosacea Diet*. This revision of the *Rosacea Diet* is at least the fourth major one and includes new chapters and information gleaned over the past year.

I have had rosacea for over twenty years, and cannot remember exactly when it was first diagnosed by a dermatologist who prescribed tetracycline. When I was a teenager I had taken tetracycline for acne off and on so I accepted the diagnosis and the treatment. If you have a skin problem, you can't have a better name for a disease like rosacea. It sounds so flowery! A significant number of people haven't heard of rosacea so when I tell them I have it, they think I must be an impressionist painter or wonder what I am talking about.

However, my face does leave an impression upon them when I have a flare-up of rosacea. Due to the number of Americans who have rosacea more people have heard about it, However, there are the side effects of tetracycline which come with taking the drug, such as sun sensitivity and upset stomach, not to mention the cost of prescription medication and visits to the doctor. But taking tetracycline along with its side effects is better than having rosacea breakouts. That is what the medical profession refers as the benefit/risk ratio in any treatment. A patient has to determine if the benefits are worth the risks, including the side effects. What do you think the long-term effects of taking tetracycline for years are? Sometime in the Eighties the dermatologist handed me a tube of Metrogel® and said I didn't have to take tetracycline anymore! I was so happy with the gel. It even worked for a while. Then I quit using the gel and the tetracycline and my rosacea seemed to go away. But as anyone with rosacea learns, it will come back. So after a move and much stress, the rosacea did return and the Metrogel® didn't seem to help this time. I tried several natural remedies since I didn't want to go back to the tetracycline or go to the dermatologist. I was not happy with the side effects. Finally after no success at home remedies and every sort of natural treatment suggested, I returned to the dermatologist who handed me a prescription for tetracycline and Metrogel® again. I asked him why the Metrogel® wasn't working alone anymore? He said that the tetracycline works along with the Metrogel® to relieve the rosacea. So for a few years I was back again with my tetracycline dosage, which worked to control rosacea. Then by accident, I discovered how to control my rosacea without tetracycline and Metrogel®. This treatment is so simple, in fact, I save the expense of dermatologist visits and prescription medication, and it does not require any special product to purchase. It simply involves controlling my eating and drinking, a diet. I also use a few non-prescription treatments that you will find out about later. Now, don't get me wrong, the tetracycline and Metrogel® work to relieve rosacea flare-ups and you can keep going to the medical doctors and taking prescription medications if you prefer. Your rosacea may be so severe that you need prescription medication for it! Whether you use prescription medication or treatment from a physician for your rosacea or use non-prescription methods the *Rosacea Diet* can help control your rosacea. And remember, there is no known cure for rosacea, only treatment to control it.[5]

---

5.   See the chapter, *Basic Rosacea Facts*

Acknowledgements

The following are acknowledged for their insight on health for which I am grateful

William Dufty, Michael R. Eades, M.D., Mary Dan Eades, M.D., H. Leighton Steward, Morrison C. Bethea, M.D., Sam S. Andrews, M.D., Luis A. Balart, M.D., Robert C. Atkins, M.D., Nicholas V. Perricone, M.D., and Geoffrey Nase, Ph.D.

Basic Rosacea Facts

What is Rosacea?

According to the International Rosacea Foundation website, "Rosacea (pronounced roh-ZAY-sha) is a relatively common, chronic skin disorder. Most people have no knowledge of this disease, including how to recognize it and what to do about it. Rosacea is the fifth most common diagnosis made by dermatologists. A rosacea cure has yet to be found and its cause is still unknown. Knowing the symptoms and finding the treatment that works for you is the best defense against the social and psychological trauma of rosacea. Its classic symptoms are patchy flushing (redness) and inflammation, particularly on the cheeks, nose, forehead, and around the mouth. It typically appears between the ages of 30 and 50 and affects more women than men.

Because the symptoms emerge slowly, rosacea may initially be mistaken for sunburn, leading to a delay in treatment. Rosacea is a hereditary; chronic (long-term) skin disorder that most often affects the nose, forehead, cheekbones, and chin (Dr. Berasques). Groups of tiny microvessels (arterioles, capillaries, and venules) close to the surface of the skin become dilated, resulting in blotchy red areas with small papules (a small, red solid elevated inflammatory skin lesion without pus) and pustules (pus-filled inflammatory bumps). The redness can come and go, but eventually it may become permanent. Furthermore, the skin tissue can swell and thicken and may be tender and sensitive to the touch. Note: Pustules are NOT pimples. Pimples have a bacterial component to their makeup and are also mainly localized in and around the hair follicles...."[1]

According to Dr. Geoffrey Nase, Ph.D., "...at the most basic level, rosacea is a disorder of the facial blood vessels. This disorder results in hyper-responsive blood vessels that dilate to numerous internal and external stimuli. This causes frequent facial flushing and skin changes such as facial redness, inflammatory papules, pustules, burning sensations and rhinophyma...."[2]

"Rosacea is a chronic, relapsing and potentially life-disruptive disorder of the facial skin...Facial redness from rosacea may appear similar to a blush or sunburn, and may be caused by flushing—when a large amount of blood flows through vessels quickly and the vessels expand under the skin to handle the flow..."[3]

Classifications of Rosacea

There are at least three ways rosacea is classified—the traditional classification, Dr. Nase's classification, and the National Rosacea Society's classification.[4]

The traditional[5] classification of rosacea involves three stages:

Stage I—Erythema (redness)
Stage II—Inflammatory papules and pustules
Stage III—Large inflammatory nodules, furunculoid infiltrations, and tissue hyperplasia

---

1. International Rosacea Foundation > http://internationalrosaceafoundation.org/
2. source > http://drnase.com/faq.htm
3. National Rosacea Society > http://rosacea.org/patients/whatis.html
4. In the booklet, *Coping With Rosacea*, National Rosacea Society, on page 13 this booklet lists the Stages of Rosacea as follows—*Early Stage, Middle Stage, and Advanced Stage.*
5. Three Stages—Plewig and Kligman Classification of Rosacea, *Acne and Rosacea*, Second Edition, 1993) source > http://internationalrosaceafoundation.org/

Dr. Geoffrey Nase, Ph.D., classifies rosacea into four[6] general stages:

Pre-Rosacea
Mild Rosacea
Moderate Rosacea
Severe Rosacea

The National Rosacea Society developed a new standard classification system that divides rosacea into four subtypes:[7]

Subtype 1: Facial Redness (erythematotelangiectatic rosacea)
Subtype 2: Bumps and Pimples (papulopustular rosacea)
Subtype 3: Skin Thickening (phymatous rosacea)
Subtype 4: Eye Irritation (ocular rosacea)

Untreated rosacea may develop into rhinophyma, which the nose has hypertrophy of the sebaceous tissue resulting in some serious disfigurement.[8]

Diagnosis and Assessment

An *International Journal of Dermatology* report indicates that "at present, there are no standard validated tools for assessing the severity of rosacea or its signs or symptoms."[9]

---

6. *Beating Rosacea Vascular, Ocular & Acne Forms, A Must-Have Guide to Understanding & Treating Rosacea,* Geoffrey Nase, Ph.D., Nase Publications, 2001, page 283, www.drnase.com

7. See footnote number 4, *Preface,* page xi

8. http://www.meddean.luc.edu/lumen/MedEd/medicine/dermatology/melton/rhinol.htm

9. *International Journal of Dermatology,* Volume 42, Issue 6, Page 444, June 2003, *Measuring the severity of rosacea: a review,* Charles E. Gessert, MD, MPH, and Joel T. M. Bamford, MD

"There are no histological, serological or other diagnostic tests for rosacea. A diagnosis of rosacea must come from your physician after a thorough examination of your signs and symptoms and a medical history."
source >
National Rosacea Society, Answer to Question 5 >
http://www.rosacea.org/patients/faq.html

What is the Cause of Rosacea?

There are many theories on what causes rosacea, but that is what they are theories. No one knows for sure what causes rosacea no matter what you have read. Geoffrey Nase, Ph.D. Microvascular Physiologist, wrote a book that is probably one of the most comprehensive work of research on rosacea published in book form to date. Dr. Nase lists possibly the longest list of some of the proposed triggers (or causes) as follows; "bacteria, yeast, mites, blood vessel damage, nerve dysfunction, systemic infection, gastrointestinal abnormalities, immune system alterations, psychological problems, liver problems, leaky intestines, collagen damage, sun damage, skin irritation, hormonal variations, stress, exercise, facial parasites, blood toxins, sebaceous gland hyperactivity, hair follicle abnormalities, stomach hyperacidity, nervous system defects, cardiovascular abnormalities, food allergies, environmental damage, etc..."[10]

Dr. Nase minimizes the above-proposed triggers stating that in "the average rosacea sufferer, these are not important in rosacea development or progression."[11] For instance, he says the H. Pylori theory is only a minimally important rosacea trigger,[12] that there is no evidence

---

10. *Beating Rosacea Vascular, Ocular & Acne Forms, A Must-Have Guide to Understanding & Treating Rosacea*, Geoffrey Nase, Ph.D., Nase Publications, 2001, page 32
11. ibid., page 288, See also pages 84–114
12. ibid., page 109, 288

that liver problems cause or worsen rosacea and that the demodex mite plays no real role in the development of rosacea 'except for the odd pustule.'[13] Dr. Nase states in his book that "rosacea is primarily a facial vascular disorder in which the affected blood vessels are functionally and structurally abnormal."[14] Further he states that rosacea "is a mysterious disorder that continues to receive very little focus by the general medical community....[and] is surrounded by confusion, unproven theories, and erroneous speculation."[15] Dr. Nase does state that "rosacea is caused by frequent facial flushing." [16] However he also states that the "exact cellular reasons are not yet fully understood." [17] He also lists nine main triggers for facial flushing and rosacea progression.[18] More information on his book can be obtained at his site >
http://www.drnase.com/

"...It can be argued that all the stigmata of rosacea are manifestations of an inflammatory process: neutrophilic dermatosis...The pathophysiology of rosacea is still a subject of controversy. Research suggests that various immune cells and inflammatory mediators play a role in the vascular, inflammatory, and hyperplasia stages of this disorder."[19]

"No one knows for certain what causes rosacea."[20]

"There are many theories but none have been proven."[21]

---

13. ibid., page 110, 114, 288
14. ibid., page 43
15. ibid., page 31, 288
16. ibid., page 284
17. ibid., page 285 (See also page 43 under the question, WHAT IS UNIQUE ABOUT ROSACEA BLOOD VESSELS?, in which Dr. Nase lists three plausible theories.)
18. ibid., page 285
19. *The Proposed Inflammatory Pathophysiology of Rosacea: Implications for Treatment,* Larry Millikan, MD source > http://groups.yahoo.com/group/rosacea-knowledge/message/1447
20. International Rosacea Foundation > http://internationalrosaceafoundation.org/

According to the National Institute of Arthritis and Musculoskeletal and Skin Diseases, National Institutes of Health, "Doctors do not know the exact cause of rosacea but believe that a combination of genetic predisposition and several types of environmental factors are related to its development. Some researchers believe that rosacea is primarily a disorder of the blood vessels, or vascular system, in which something causes blood vessels to swell, resulting in flushing and redness.

A tiny organism called Demodex folliculorum, a mite that lives in facial hair follicles, may be involved. Some researchers believe that these mites clog the sebaceous gland openings, leading to inflammation. Other investigators have shown a possible link between rosacea and Helicobacter pylori, a bacterium that causes infection in the gastrointestinal system. Also, some research has suggested that the immune system may play a role in the development of rosacea in some people...."[22]

"The exact cause of rosacea is unknown, although several theories exist. One theory of rosacea's origin is that the disease may be a component of a more generalized disorder of the blood vessels, which could explain why rosacea sufferers have a tendency to flush. Another theory is that changes in normal skin bacteria or infection of the stomach by Helicobacter pylori may play a role. Other theories suggest that the condition is caused by microscopic skin mites (Demodex), fungus, a malfunction of the connective tissue under the skin or even psychological factors. None of these possibilities has been proven."[23]

---

21.   *Rosacea—What You should Know*, page 7, Galderma Laboratories, Inc.
22.   source of article—http://www.nih.gov/niams/healthinfo/rosacea.htm
23.   National Rosacea Society source > http://www.rosacea.org/patients/faq.html

"The cause of rosacea is unknown, but it is commonly thought to be of vascular origin because of a clinical association with flushing, development of telangiectasia and tissue swelling, and ultimately, tissue proliferation and rhinophyma (enlargement of the nose)."[24]

"...Pathogenesis [of rosacea] is not clearly understood...'[25]

"...Currently, neither a specific cause nor a laboratory indicator of rosacea has been suggested...."[26]

"...All the treatment [of rosacea] seems to go towards treating the symptoms only, because the cause is unknown..."[27]

There is evidence that the immune system may be involved in rosaceans.[28]

Can Rosacea Be Cured?

"Rosacea can't be cured..."[29]

"Just as there is no cure for the common cold, there is no cure for rosacea..."[30]

---

24. Postgraduate Medicine source of article > http://www.postgradmed.com/issues/ 1999/02_99/millikan.htm

25. Thissen MR, Neumann HA., Academisch Ziekenhuis—source of article > http://www.ncbi.nlm.nih.gov:80/entrez/ query.fcgi?cmd=Retrieve&db=PubMed&list_uids=11582639&dopt=Abstract

26. *Rosacea: current thoughts on origin.* Bamford JT., Department of Family Practice and Community Health, University of Minnesota-Duluth Medical School, MN, USA. Jbamford@smdc.org—source of article > http://www.ncbi.nlm.nih.gov:80/entrez/ query.fcgi?cmd=Retrieve&db=PubMed&list_uids=11594675&dopt=Abstract

27. A nurse's insightful comment on the cause of rosacea > http://groups.yahoo.com/group/rosacea-support/message/34090?threaded=1

"The condition rarely reverses itself and may last for years...."[31]

"...A variety of treatments exist that can eliminate pustules, but no therapy is highly effective in eliminating the vascular flushing associated with rosacea...."[32]

Can Rosacea Be Treated or Controlled?

"Rosacea can't be cured, but it can be controlled."[33]

"...Effective treatment along with changes in lifestyle can help to control and manage the discomfort of this condition..."[34]

"While there is no cure for rosacea, medical therapy is available to control or reverse its signs and symptoms. Individuals who suspect they

28. **Involvement of immune mechanisms in the pathogenesis of rosacea.**
1: Br J Dermatol 1982 Aug; 107(2): 203–8 Related Articles, Books, Manna V, Marks R, Holt P.
Twenty-five patients with rosacea were compared with twenty-five control subjects for previous medical history and tests of immune function. Rosacea patients were found to have a higher incidence of disorders of the autoimmune type and were significantly more difficult to sensitize to DNCB than the controls. In addition, twelve of the rosacea patients and eleven other rosacea patients had biopsies which were examined by the direct immunofluorescence technique. In only five was the test negative. In the remainder deposits of IgM and/or IgG and/or complement were found at the dermo-epidermal junction and/or in the dermal collagen. Serum from the rosacea patients was also examined by the indirect technique and in six cases a circulating antinuclear antibody of IgM type was found. It is suggested that altered immune function plays a significant role in the pathogenesis of the disease.
PMID: 6213254 [PubMed—indexed for MEDLINE]
source > http://www.ncbi.nlm.nih.gov/htbin-post/Entrez/query?uid=6213254&form=6&db=m&Dopt=b
29. *Rosacea—What You Should Know*, page 3, Galderma Laboratories, Inc., See also *Coping With Rosacea*, National Rosacea Society, page 1, "Rosacea cannot be cured..."

may have rosacea are urged to see a dermatologist for diagnosis and appropriate treatment."[35]

"Although rosacea is incurable, its progress can be controlled and even halted through medical therapy and lifestyle modification..."[36]

It cannot be overemphasized that you need a diagnosis from a physician if you have rosacea (see the chapter, *Physician Treatment*). Rosacea may be misdiagnosed for many other diseases[37] and there is 'mass confusion over rosacea and its treatment.'[38]

Finding a physician who is up to date with the latest rosacea treatment is the trick. If you think that you have rosacea and have self-diagnosed yourself you may be wrong. You really need to consider seriously seeing a physician to rule out other diseases or find out if you also have another disease even if you have rosacea. You may have several other

---

30.   International Rosacea Foundation, http://internationalrosaceafoundation.org/summary.html

31.   American Academy of Dermatology, http://www.aad.org/pamphlets/rosacea.html

32.   *Rosacea*, Zuber TJ, Saginaw Cooperative Hospitals, Inc. Department of Family Practice, Michigan State University and Aleda E. Lutz Veterans Administration Medical Center, Saginaw, Michigan, source > http://www.ncbi.nlm.nih.gov:80/entrez/query.fcgi?cmd=Retrieve&db=PubMed&list_uids=10815045&dopt=Abstract

33.   See footnote 29

34.   International Rosacea Foundation, http://internationalrosaceafoundation.org/summary.html

35.   National Rosacea Society source > http://www.rosacea.org/patients/whatis.html

36.   *Postgraduate Medicine*, source of article—http://www.postgradmed.com/issues/1999/02_99/millikan.htm

37.   A partial list of diseases misdiagnosed for rosacea can be found at the following url > http://www.rosaceans.com/html/other.html
(Also see the chapter, *Physician Treatment*, under the subheading, Rosacea May Be Misdiagnosed for other Diseases)

diseases along with your rosacea. Having a competent physician is a must have to diagnose what you may have. It is not unheard of to get a second or third opinion since what is on your face may or may not be rosacea or something else (see the chapter, *Physician Treatment*).

Gathering information on rosacea and doing your own research is also a must. Relying solely on your physician is no substitute for understanding your rosacea. Everyone who has rosacea is different. The more information you can gather will help you sort out all this confusion and bring you satisfaction since you have done your homework. My website is dedicated to gather all the commercial and non-commercial information on rosacea into one website. If you find something I am not aware about please email me so I can post it.

http://www.rosacea-diet.com

---

38. *Beating Rosacea Vascular, Ocular & Acne Forms, A Must-Have Guide to Understanding & Treating Rosacea*, Geoffrey Nase, Ph.D., Nase Publications, 2001, page 32

Diet and Rosacea

There are so many diets out there that you may wonder how this diet could be any help for your rosacea. The *Rosacea Diet* is just for **thirty days** to prove that you can control your rosacea. This diet may seem extreme to you since it may be a radical change from your lifestyle. If you actually have the will power to follow this diet for thirty days you will see improvement in controlling your rosacea. There are hundreds of users who have found it works. Unlike other diets, the *Rosacea Diet* is only for thirty days. After the thirty days you can go back to eating whatever you want. You will benefit by knowing the *Rosacea Diet* helps control your rosacea and can either go back on it or modify it any way you want, depending on your rosacea. All diets have to juggle the three basic food groups—carbohydrate, protein and fat. Most diets avoid or discourage fat. Rarely does anyone advocate a high fat diet. The *Rosacea Diet* encourages you to not worry about fat during the thirty days. Be assured that thirty days not worrying about fat in your diet is in no way a health risk. The *Rosacea Diet* is not a high fat diet so you don't have to worry about that either. More on fat will be discussed later. That leaves just two remaining food groups. Diets are either a high protein or a high carbohydrate or a so-called 'balanced food group' diet. High complex carbohydrate diets have been the rage for many years, while the high protein diets have come and gone and returned in recent popularity. The *diet authorities* usually stick to the balanced basic food group approach, the U.S. Department of Agriculture's (USDA) Food Guide Pyramid. There are other pyramids suggested, such as, the Mediterranean Diet Pyramid, the Asian Diet Pyramid, and the Latin American Diet Pyramid which are all meant to help you. I have a chapter on pyramids that you will enjoy. You obviously have your own diet beliefs and I respect that. I know you have some cherished beliefs about you current diet. But remember the reason you are reading the *Rosacea Diet*, **you are a rosacean. You have rosacea.** You want to control your rosacea because you know, deep down inside you that something you are eating or drinking is triggering your rosacea and you know it. The *diet authorities* haven't suggested what it is, nor your doctor so that is why you bought this book. You obviously are reading this book hoping that you can discover what to eat and drink to control your rosacea. Hundreds of users have found the *Rosacea Diet* does control rosacea. **So, for thirty days let all your diet beliefs disappear.** Can you just let your cherished diet beliefs go for thirty days? You can always return to your diet beliefs at the end of this thirty-day period and eat whatever you want! **Thirty Days**…*Rosacea Diet*. I repeat myself so you will get the point.

The Diet Authority

You have heard of the two most controversial subjects—religion and politics, right? There is a third, diet. You don't think so? These three subjects have been debated as far back as the Garden of Eden when a diet involved religion and sovereignty. You don't think diet is controversial? Why are there so many diet books? Try discussing diet with your friends, family or strangers and note the reaction. Everyone is a *diet authority*. Everyone knows what *you* should eat or what *you* shouldn't eat. Discussing what to eat and drink involves human emotion. Ask a vegetarian to explain tofu to a meat eater. Have fun storming the castle![1]

The big question is, 'what is the *correct* diet? And who is to say what is the correct diet? By what authority does any person or organization have to say what is the correct diet? For rosaceans this is important since there are all sorts of authorities giving you food and beverage trigger lists with offending food and drink! Even if the highest authority you can think of told you what to eat and drink, would you follow the diet suggested? Adam and Eve had a problem with the *diet authority*. Most people ignore the 'correct diet' since everyone wants to make their own decision as to what to eat and drink. And choosing what to eat and drink is a basic human right so universally accepted that it is not in any Bill of Rights or Universal Declaration of Human Rights. It

---

1. "…The controversial nature of vegetarianism—a nutritional issue always able to trigger a crossfire of debate—is acknowledged in our pages by two chapters with differing views on the subject…."—*The Cambridge World History of Food* by Kenneth F. Kiple & Kriemhild Conee Ornelee published by Cambridge University Press, http://www.cup.org/books/kiple/default.htm

is simply understood by everyone that an adult can choose whatever he or she wants to eat and drink without impunity or restrictions.

An example of a people who ignore a *diet authority* is in the USA. Most Americans who eat 'the average American diet' have largely ignored the USDA's Food Guide Pyramid created in 1992. *Newsweek*[2] magazine describes this diet as "…with a cherry on top. Sweets and meats are a bigger draw than healthful fruits and vegetables." No one likes a food cop. What if the government forced everyone to eat the Food Guide Pyramid or some other *authorized* diet? Diet should be added to the list following religion and politics as the third most controversial subject. This book will add to the controversy because I have no initials behind my name, like M.D., Ph.D., or whatever. I am not a nutritionist. I am simply an average American who discovered what helps to lose weight, feel healthier, and control my rosacea. There are thousands of diet books—the sheer number of them proves there is controversy. The more popular the diet book is the more controversy it brings. The browbeating, mud slinging, and criticism against and among diet book writers, critics, and *diet authorities* are cornucopian. A diet for rosaceans is no exception.

Michael Fumento has a website[3] discussing this controversy and wrote an interesting article entitled, *Living Off the Fat of the Land: The Only People Benefiting From Diet Books are the Authors* (*Washington Monthly*, Jan-Feb 18). In this article he wrote about the first diet guru, appearing more than a century ago, William Banting, who actually got his diet from the British ear surgeon William Harvey. Banting lost weight on this diet and later published the diet as *Banting's Letter on Corpulence*. Since Banting's background wasn't in health, but rather he was an undertaker, this established the precedent that anyone can write a diet book. This revision of my book is based on research and the user feed-

---

2.   *Newsweek*, January 20, 2003, p.52
3.   http://www.fumento.com

back from users over a period of more than four years. I am basically self-taught and learned most of my nutrition on health from Carol Ann Rinzler's book[4] and other books I mention. I was an EMT for about ten years but that doesn't even get me a cup of coffee. My certification expired years ago.

My belief is that wisdom is proved righteous by its works. The *Rosacea Diet* works. You will decide for yourself. That is what this chapter is about. Do you think that thirty-days on my diet poses any health risks? No, that is not possible. It is important that you understand that this diet is for thirty days. After that you decide what you want to do with this diet.

The *Rosacea Diet* after the thirty days *may* become to you a way of thinking and a lifestyle. Who is the authority to tell you what to eat and drink? Am I? You have got to be kidding. I can't convince you what to eat and drink. Only you can decide this for yourself, since it a basic human right understood universally that you decide what to eat and drink for yourself.

So why would you bother to read a book telling you what to eat and drink? Again, as I said before, you are a rosacean. Controlling your rosacea with diet is the goal. I am confident the *Rosacea Diet* can change the way you think about food and drink and will help you control your rosacea. Hundreds of user feedback reports have established this diet works to control rosacea. The results are conclusive. Diet controls rosacea.

You will hear about 30 days, 30 grams and many other things repetitively. I learned over the past few years that when people read my book they asked me repetitive questions so my reaction is to follow the same

---

4.   *Nutrition for Dummies*, Carol Ann Rinzler, 1997, IDG Books Worldwide, Inc.

pattern and be repetitive in my writing to prevent frequently asked questions. This revision is no exception to the repetition.

You may not have given much thought about why you eat the way you do, but you obviously are thinking about it now. Stop and think for a moment about your current diet. Your mother (or whoever fed you in childhood) made choices you make now. You trusted Mom (or whoever fed you) and so how can Mom be wrong about diet? This is not to say that Mom did not have your best interest at heart. The point is that you probably were influenced to choose the food and drink that is on your current diet and this also has an emotional impact on your life. Food is such a controversial subject since what we eat and drink has an emotional impact on our lives. Food and drink should impact our emotional state for the better. At a party the food and drink can play such an important emotional impact on the event as to whether it is successful or not. Whatever emotional state we are in, whether happy, sad, or under stress, food has such a tremendous emotional impact on us. Try eating or drinking with an enemy of yours? The way we respond to life stresses is so deeply psychologically rooted in us that sometimes we don't realize what we are doing to ourselves. Remember the saying, *you are what you eat*? You are also what your mom gave you to eat. Mom learned how to eat and drink from her mother and so on. So what is the point? The *diet authority* that first influenced you to eat was Mom or you may have been impacted by another *diet authority* or diet book. Is it possible that Mom has been wrong about diet? Could your Mom have been influenced to give you food that isn't healthy for you or is triggering your rosacea? How could Mom be wrong? How can there be so many diet books with so many different approaches from so many different *diet authorities* especially when you consider there are only three basic food groups and every diet just juggles the three around? Why is there so much controversy?

It has been said that, "uncertainties still cloud our understanding of the relation between diet and health."[5] Yet we know there is a relationship between diet and health. So lets take a history lesson with food, a lesson you haven't thought about till now. The human race has not been eating and drinking the same way since the beginning. A change started to occur around 1700, the beginning of the eighteenth century. What am I talking about?

For millenniums mankind generally ate fruit, vegetables, dairy, eggs, grains, seafood, fish, fowl, and meats. Anthropologically speaking, a big change in diet started to occur just a few hundred years ago resulting in a dramatic change in diet that has effected the choices you and your Mom are making in food and drink. This change effected *diet authorities* in the Twentieth Century and dramatically changed the diet mankind eats today. Diet books and *diet authorities* have been impacted by what happened. What happened? The sugar industry began to emerge with great economic power. I have arbitrarily chosen the beginning of the Eighteenth Century as the start of the *'Sugar Age'* since statistics show that the average Englishman ate 4 pounds of sugar a year at this point and before this very little consumption of sugar is known.

Later the sugar industry became part of the processed food industry of the twentieth century. The processed food industry has a tremendous impact on a major portion of the planet economically thus effecting your choice of food and drink especially with the advent of globalization. This is not to say that the processed food industry is intrinsically bad. Certainly having food and drink processed has many advantages. It is nice to see food protected in clear plastic wrap or nice package. Having safe food and drink clean and free from contaminates is wonderful. Having food processed makes obtaining it easier and quicker for

5.   *Scientific American*, January 2003, *Rebuilding the Food Guide Pyramid*, Walter C. Willett and Meir J. Stampfer

billions of people. The main advantage usually is that the price of food processed by an industry is cheaper than food we could grow ourselves, not to mention the convenience. Besides, in this system who has the time or ability to grow or raise their own food? There are no doubt other good things to say about the processed food industry. But the choice you make as to what you eat and drink is certainly influenced by this industry probably more than you may have thought. Could there be something in the processed food industry that may be causing obesity, other health problems or a factor in your rosacea? How much influence do you think the processed food industry has on you or your Mom?

Since the last century the *'diet authorities'* have pointed to **fat** as the culprit[6] for health problems. Hence, a plethora of fat free or low fat diets and products have been offered, and the processed food industry responded with low fat (or without fat) food and drink. The advertising of these products influences millions, if not billions. Yet when you look at the results over the last century obesity has risen particularly since 1992. In the developed world obese people are at a record high despite what the *'diet authorities'* have said about the dangers of eating too much fat. A Worldwatch Institute study reveals that the overfed now equals the underfed. Some 1.2 billion people are underfed and hungry and an equal number or more now eat too much. *The New York Times* commented on this study by saying,

> "The number of overweight people in the world now rivals the number of hungry, underfed people."

---

6.   "The belief that fat is the dietary bad guy is about as close to universal as any idea in America."—*The World's Biggest Fad Diet* by Dean Esmay source > http://www.survivediabetes.com/lowfat.html

The Worldwatch Institute's *State of the World 2000* states,

> "Half the world's people, both rich and poor, are medically mal-
> nourished, suffering from either obesity or from diets with inade-
> quate calories, vitamins, or minerals. A whopping 55 percent of
> American adults are overweight."

This paradox doesn't make any sense. As the processed food industry
of the developed world makes inroads into the underdeveloped world
the result is a diet producing obesity. Rosacea during this same period
has increased dramatically worldwide. The current number of Americans with rosacea is over 14 million. In England the rosaceans are estimated to be somewhere between 8 to 10 million. In Canada the
number of rosaceans is estimated to be 4 to 6 million. This gives you
an idea of the global rosacean population.

What does the underdeveloped people of the world die of? Primarily
the cause of death is infectious diseases due to malnutrition and poor
hygiene. What is the primary cause of death in the developed world?
The cause is primarily what the World Health Organization classifies
as "Noncommunicable Conditions" which include vascular disorders
(such as heart disease, stroke and diabetes) and all cancers. Diet is a factor in these deaths. What accounts for the obesity in the developed
world? While fat has been the accused culprit in the minds of many,
there is another culprit emerging as the culprit, *sugar*.

A growing number of people have discovered that sugar is the cause of
obesity. How is this possible? Simply, *excess sugar in the diet is converted
to fat*. It is an undisputed fact that sugar is a factor in obesity. The processed food industry uses sugar in a large percentage of the food and
drink prepared and sold to the world. Most people in the world are
ignorant of this or don't care. Historically sugar's health problems have
either been minimized or dismissed by the 'diet authorities' and the
processed food industry. Coupled with the fast food industry which

also uses sugar in its food and drink the results are that 55% of American adults are overweight and the rest of the developed world is trying to catch up to the Americans in obesity. Some figures indicate that the number of obese Americans is even higher. As the processed food industry moves into underdeveloped countries obesity rises and along with it rises in vascular disorders and cancers which shows the influence this industry has on people's choices.

Rosacea is a vascular disorder. Diet no doubt is a factor in the development of rosacea just as diet is a factor in all other vascular disorders, cancers and obesity.

Why is sugar used in such large percentages in the processed food industry? Basically it is cheap to produce, yields higher profit, makes the food taste better, and is addictive. As Sidney W. Mintz writes in his book, *Sweetness and Power—The Place of Sugar in Modern History,*[7] on pages 190–192,

> "Per hectare (2.7 acres), sugar cane yields, under optimum conditions, about twenty tons of dry material, some half of which is in the form of sugar usable as food or feed; the other ten tons of cane 'trash,' or bagasse, is usable as fuel and for the manufacture of paper products, building materials, and furfuraldehyde (a liquid aldehyde used in manufacturing nylon and resins, and as a solvent)...An acre of good subtropical land will now produce more than eight million calories in sugar, beyond the other products it yields...antisaccarites are compelled to recognize sugar's appeal on grounds of taste, energy economy, relative cost, and calories—an appeal sugar manufacturers clearly recognize, and which their political, professorial, and professional supporters push vigorously."

7.   *Sweetness and Power—The Place of Sugar in Modern History,* Sidney W. Mintz, 1985, Penguin Books

Professor Mintz writes on page 192,

> "Where the need for calories, let alone other food values, is a serious problem, sucrose may not be a good nutritional answer (in large quantities, I think it is a terrible one); but circumstances early made it, and have kept it, what looks like a good economic answer. When one adds to this the remarkable energy-transforming nature of plants like sugar cane and maize—even at high levels of human input in the form of fertilizers, cultivation, etc., the solar-energy input is approximately 90 percent of the total energy consumed in producing a usable food—the appeal of sucrose as a solution to food problems becomes almost irresistible."

Professor Mintz's book is a remarkable anthropological insight into the power of the sugar industry and the change sugar has made on mankind in the relatively short period of just the last few centuries. Westernization, modernization, industrialization, globalization or the modern development of the world cannot be fully understood historically or anthropologically without sucrose power as a factor to consider. The power of the sugar industry is tremendous. Most sugar in the world has traditionally or historically been the sucrose from sugar cane or sugar beets. Now high fructose corn syrup (HFCS) has exceeded the production of sugar cane or sugar beet sucrose. This billion-dollar sugar industry whether made from sucrose or high fructose corn syrup has had tremendous impact on your diet. Can you imagine the economic impact a company like Coca-Cola ® has on mankind in selling its product? That is just one company pushing sugar not only in the developed world but now in practically every country of the underdeveloped world. And does Coke ® know how to sell its product? Is it successful? A thirsty, sugar-loving people of the world love Coke ® because of the advertising and promotion of this product, not to mention its wonderful taste[8]. I am simply using this example to help you see the impact of the economic power of sugar. So many major corpo-

---

8. It would be nice if Diet Coke ® would use Stevia as a sugar substitute

rations use sugar or high fructose corn syrup. When *Coca-Cola* ®
changed from sucrose to high fructose corn syrup this had a major
impact why HFCS has now become the largest sugar processed and
consumed.

So your choices as to food and drink have been impacted to a large
degree to eat sugar in greater quantities. At the turn of the Eighteenth
Century (1700) the average Englishman ate four (4) pounds of sugar a
year. By the turn of the Nineteenth Century (1800) it had risen to 18
pounds a year (*Sweetness and Power*, page 67). However, the United
States by 1880–8 was consuming 38 pounds of sucrose per person per
year, the second highest consumer just under the British (Sweetness
and Power, page 188). When the Twentieth Century rolled around the
British and the Americans were neck and neck since the per-capita figure for the first time rose above 90 pounds per person. (*Sweetness and
Power*, page 143) From then till 1996 the figures keep rising to 149
pounds[9] per person in the USA! These figures are similar in European
countries with the English and the Icelandic the largest consumers of
sugar in a world that competes to be in first place in sugar consumption. What this means is that the production and consumption of
sugar has increased dramatically only in the last two to three hundred
years! You and your Mom have been eating quite differently than your
ancestors that lived before the *Sugar Age*.

An interesting tidbit is that at the beginning of the twentieth century
most sugar consumed was purchased by itself and then added to food.
The consumer added sugar to what was consumed. By the end of the
century most sugar consumed is now already added in food and drink
processed. Since most people purchase small amounts of sugar by itself
a consumer may be mislead into thinking that very little sugar is being

---

9.   *Sugar Busters!* by H. Leighton Steward, Dr. Morrison C. Bethea, Dr. Samued
      Dr. Luis A Balart, 1995, *Sugar Busters!*, LLC, Figure 2, page 43

consumed. However the facts show that the average consumer is eating tremendous amounts of sugar from processed food and drink.

While sucrose has historically been the main focus of the sugar industry, there is a growing industry of alternative sugars, such as high fructose corn syrup, sugar substitutes and other sugars. The list of sugars is massive (see the chapter *Sugars to Avoid*). High Fructose Corn Syrup (HFCS) has now reached greater production than sucrose made from either sugar cane or beets. Mintz writes on page 73 of his book that this consumption of sugar "may be enough to say that probably no other food in world history has had a comparable performance." Two exhaustive works on food[10] both give a significant amount of discussion on sugar and desserts. *The Cambridge World History of Food* by Kenneth F. Kiple & Kriemhild Conee Ornelee has been called the 'food book of the millennium' by *Science Magazine*. Kipple and Ornelle state in their book,

"...for those seeking a "heart-healthy" diet....wonder that despite their increasing longevity, many people in the developed world have become abruptly and acutely anxious about what they do and do not put in their mouths....Nor are developing-world peoples so likely as those in the developed world to survive the nutritional disorders that seem to be legacies of our hunter-gatherer past. Diabetes (which may be the result of a "thrifty" gene for carbohydrate metabolism) is one of these diseases, and hypertension may be another; still others are doubtless concealed among a group of food allergies, sensitivities, and intolerances that have only recently begun to receive the attention they deserve..."[11]

10. *The Cambridge World History of Food* by Kenneth F. Kiple & Kriemhild Conee Ornelee, Cambridge University Press > http://www.cup.org/books/kiple/default.htm
The Oxford Companion to Food by Alan Davidson, Oxford University Press 1999
11. http://www.cup.org/books/kiple/default.htm

The above quote helps to understand everyone's concern about diet. The 'sensitivities' and 'intolerances' may include not only diabetes but also rosacea! You would think that nutritionists and medical authorities (who are *diet authorities*) would be in agreement on what the *perfect* diet should be. When you bring the processed food industry into the picture, economics becomes the factor in this disunity. The *diet authorities* are impacted by this industry. Capitalism, greed, emotions, nutrition and basic human rights are in a tangled mess when it comes to deciding what factors influence your choice of food and drink.

The *Newsweek* magazine article, *Stacking up the Perfect Diet*,[12] mentions "millions of Americans who desperately want to change their unhealthy ways, but can't quite get started." On page 6 of this magazine it states,

> "The federal government has long tried to distill the best science on diet and health. But commercial pressures and bureaucratic obstacles have often clouded the results. The USDA's famous Food Guide Pyramid, first published in 1992, is now widely viewed as flawed. 'The pyramid is a disaster,' says K. Dun Gifford of Oldways, a non-profit think tank based in Boston. 'The American epidemic of obesity is the proof that it hasn't worked. Period. Amen.'"

The economic pressure of the processed food industry on Americans, as well as on the rest of the world is summed up nicely on page 51 of this same magazine:

> "A second point of consensus is that vegetables should be eaten in abundance. There isn't a diet guru who denies their virtues. Heart doctors endorse them, cancer doctors endorse them, the USDA endorses them, and even the low-carb king Dr. Robert Atkins endorses them. Unfortunately, no one can afford to promote spinach or bell peppers the way snackmakers promote their goods.

---

12. *Newsweek*, January 20, 2003

McDonald's spent $1.1 billion on advertising in 2001. That same year the budget for the governments' pro-vegetable '5 a Day for Better Health' program was 1.1 *million*. Not surprisingly, only 23 percent of U.S. adults were meeting the five-a-day target at last count."

Mom and the processed food industry have conditioned you to eat and drink the 'average American diet' and now you want to change your diet? When Mom gave you ice cream, apple pie and a *Coke* ® you felt happy and trusted Mom. She was giving you comfort. Now you want to change your diet? This is not going to be easy. You have to be motivated. Hopefully this book will be the motivating factor. The motivation is short term to prove you can control your rosacea with diet. In the long term you will have to decide what to do with your diet. You may decide from this experience to make a dramatic life style diet change!

Getting back to the question, 'Who is the Diet Authority?" **The diet authority is you**. You can read all the diet books on the planet for information or listen to the 'food cops' but you still decide what to eat and drink. As long as there is choice in the food and drink available, *you are the diet authority*. Maybe soylent green[13] will be all that is available but for now you have a choice. However, the emotional impact when Mom, a 'food cop,' a friend or the processed food industry offers you food or drink is very deep. Remember that **you are the diet authority.**

---

13. *Soylent Green* (1973) is a film directed by Richard Fleischer based on a novel by Harry Harrison (Make Room! Make Room!) starring Charlton Heston, screenplay by Harry Harrison and Stanley R. Greenberg—if you haven't seen the film, I rate it a two star film worth watching. You will never forget it once you see it.

A Simple Method to Control Rosacea

One way that has proved effective to control rosacea is to visit a dermatologist like I did for many years and get prescription medication which controls rosacea and is effective in treating rosacea symptoms. There is no known cure for rosacea, only treatment to control it.[1] However, I kept thinking that rosacea had something to do with what I was eating, since after eating certain foods I would break out with rosacea usually the next day, sometimes the same day! You probably notice yourself after eating certain foods, breaking out with rosacea, too. I avoided certain food and drink only to find the symptoms return. There seemed to be no logical pattern to the foods or drinks I avoided since I kept breaking out with rosacea no matter what I tried. I resorted to taking the tetracycline with all its side effects for many years and putting Metrogel® on my face, which seemed at the time to be the only alternative. But I worried about the long-term effects of the tetracycline and longed for a way to avoid rosacea flare-ups without taking prescription medications. I was on the right track that something I was eating triggered the rosacea, but was unsuccessful in discovering what to avoid. That was because I didn't know what the real culprit is that triggers rosacea in the food and drink I was consuming.

Then one day in 1998, my wife decided to read *Sugar Blues* by William Dufty, Warner Books, Inc, for her own reasons, and encouraged me to read it as well. Thanks to her and Mr. Dufty I was moved to avoid sugar[2] in my diet and very soon discovered sugar was the culprit.

---

1.   See the chapter, *Basic Rosacea Facts*

Sugar, that is, refined sugar [sucrose], seems to be the catalyst for rosacea. Usually when I refer to sugar I am talking about refined sugar or sucrose, which is processed into a white crystal (you will realize soon that all carbohydrate is simply different units of sugar if you didn't know!). Also I found that a diet high in natural sugar or a high carbohydrate diet could trigger rosacea. The results were significant. My face cleared up! My personal theory from this experience is that eating too much sugar in any form, whether sucrose or whatever type sugar in the diet along with processed foods over the years taxes the pancreas or other organs, like the liver. This may upset the immune system hormonal balance causing diseases such as rosacea or other vascular disorders. There is evidence that sugar reduces the body's immune system to heal.[3] There is also evidence that rosacea sufferers may have immune system damage.[4] Most natural doctors and a few medical doctors agree that sugar is toxic.[5] There is one source on the world wide web that I am aware of that discovered that sugar is the culprit for acne[6] and there are probably others without a doubt. Rosacea-LTD III skincare products include instructions for the users of these products to avoid sugar and a high carbohydrate diet. This is a quote taken from the Rosacea LTD-III website,[7]

---

2.   See the chapter, *Sugars to Avoid*

3.   http://www.bcn.net/~stoll/sugarimm.html

4.   See footnote number 28 in the chapter, *Basic Rosacea Facts*, page 8

5.   ***Sugar Busters!*** by H. Leighton Steward, Dr. Morrison C. Bethea, Dr. Samuel S. Andrews, and Dr. Luis A Balart, 1995, *Sugar Busters!*, LLC, Figure 2, page 43 shows a graph that in 1994 the total refined sugar consumption per person per year in the USA was 149 pounds—How much did you consume over your life that has damaged your body resulting in rosacea and who knows what other diseases? On page 17 of the same publication you need to be convinced what the authors state, that "**SUGAR IS TOXIC!**" Three of the writers of this book are medical doctors and they have not lost their license for stating that sugar is toxic. These doctors are brave and should be commended for publishing this fact.

6.   http://www.thiele.fptoday.com/ta/acnehome.htm

7.   http://www.rosacea-ltd.com/lifestyle.php3

"…Rosacea redness or vascular dilation is partially caused by high calorie carbohydrate (pastas, breads) and sugar spiking from all sweet foods. Just remember kids having a sugar high and bouncing off the walls due to energy available. So think of things that give you a high burn rate, high energy, or foods that would most likely add fat to your body, and you would be identifying the worst culprits."

The International Rosacea Foundation says on its LIFESTYLE RECOMMENDATIONS page[8] on its website,

"…Rosacea redness is partially caused by high calorie carbohydrate (pastas, breads) and sugar spiking from all sweet foods. So think of things that give you a high burn rate, high energy, or foods that would most likely add fat to your body, and you would be identifying the worst culprits…"

More will continue to understand the sugar—high carbohydrate trigger factor and someday the National Rosacea Society may add sugar to their 'official' food trigger list.

Glucose and oxygen are the fuel of our body cells. You should realize that it is not necessary to obtain glucose from a diet high in sucrose or carbohydrate contrary to popular opinion. Glucose can be obtained from a high protein diet and carbohydrate with a low glycemic index. More on this is discussed later in a chapter called, *Protein Synthesis and Gluconeogenesis*.

Since there is no known cause for rosacea at present[9], only theories, my theory is just as valid. Whether anyone will research my theory in a multi-center, double blind, placebo-controlled, clinical trial study remains to be seen, but there is continuing research on rosacea. The

---

8.   http://internationalrosaceafoundation.org/lifestyle_recommendations.html
9.   See the chapter, *Rosacea Basic Facts*

National Rosacea Society may someday use research money on this theory. But for now all treatments only work on the symptoms, not the cause. The *Rosacea Diet* cannot cure your rosacea but it has proven effective in controlling rosacea as another method or treatment for many rosacea sufferers. There is enough evidence from current users to establish this, which you will read about later, in the chapter, Frequently *Asked Question*. Many have had excellent results following the *Rosacea Diet*, which continues to be improved with user feedback. This revision is largely due to user feedback. The *Rosacea Diet* Users Support Group at yahoo groups, established August 27, 2001, has a growing membership which you may join, making this group an ideal clinical study if some prestigious name or organization ever desires to spend research dollars on it. But even if a multi-center, double-blind, placebo-controlled, clinical trial study actually came to the conclusion that sugar and a diet high in carbohydrate are trigger factors in rosacea, do you think most rosaceans would change their eating and drinking habits? What do you think? Only a minority of rosaceans will alter their lifestyle diet to control their rosacea, while the majority will continue to eat sugar, starches and a high carbohydrate diet using some other way to control their rosacea.

Would my dermatologist tell me to avoid sugar? He never mentioned it. If he did, why would I need to go back to him if I followed his advice? You have probably been told by your dentist to avoid sugar because every dentist knows that sugar is the culprit for your cavities. The dentist also knows that patients won't quit eating sugar and will return to have their cavities filled, so dentists usually tell their patients to avoid sugar and brush their teeth after eating. Now think about this: it is an established fact that sugar is one of the primary causes of cavities in your teeth. Do you think that is the ONLY effect on our body from eating and drinking sugar? Could sugar also be a cause of vascular diseases or other health problems in our bodies? Could rosacea be a symptom of sugar toxicity or a factor in the cause of the disease? Sugar is also connected to obesity. Do you really think that sugar is harmless? Sugar is **toxic** and should be removed from every rosacean's diet.

Whether the dermatologist knows the connection sugar has with rosacea is a question you can ask. Very few medical authorities recognize that sugar is a rosacea trigger. The National Rosacea Society has yet to mention sugar as a trigger, but in time may include sugar and a high carbohydrate diet as a trigger factor. Dr. Nase, the 'rosacea evangelist,' does mention sugar on page 101 of his book, *Beating Rosacea—Vascular, Ocular & Acne Forms*, which says:

> "Eating large amounts of simple sugars (i.e., chocolates, syrups and food stuffs that contain large concentrations of fructose, sucrose, and maltose) can cause glucose levels in the blood stream to rise quickly and trigger skin flushing."

Dr. Nase and I have corresponded over the past year by email.

Nicholas V. Perricone, M.D., has books on how to have healthy skin and offers a number of skin care products. He also advocates a diet eating foods low in the glycemic index, avoiding refined and packaged sugar, drinking plenty of water, taking his suggested supplements, and eating fish protein. His two more popular books are *The Wrinkle Cure* and *The Perricone Prescription*. He is a licensed dermatologist. In one of his news letters, *Dr. Perricone Skin Science Update Newsletter*, he quotes some research done by the American Diabetes Association as follows,

> "…The results of several related studies presented at the June, 2002 meeting of the American Diabetes Association confirm my own finding that high-glycemic carbohydrate—sugars and starchy foods such as pasta, potatoes, and bread—cause an inflammatory response that accelerates aging and contributes to a variety of diseases (heart disease, some types of cancer, arthritis, Alzheimer's, etc.). In addition, one of the studies showed that the antioxidant vitamins E and C block this inflammatory response. The results of

the new studies support the conclusions of a prior study showing that dietary sugars increase blood levels of free radicals and pro-inflammatory enzymes to a greater degree than foods that are high in fat or protein…"

In his book, *The Wrinkle Cure*, (Warner Books) Dr. Perricone states on page 104,

> "When you consume carbohydrate, your blood sugar begins to rise and insulin is secreted by your pancreas to keep that sugar under control. The problem is that the release of insulin pushes your cellular metabolism into a mode in which it produces inflammatory chemicals….
> This whole process is very nicely described by Barry Sears, M.D., in his book *Enter the Zone* (HarperCollins, 1995). Dr. Sears explains that insulin, in high levels, tends to create chemicals in the body that encourage inflammation. The result is not only prematurely aged skin, but also degenerative diseases such as heart disease, cancer, Alzheimer's and many other illnesses.
> The best way to be sure that your insulin levels are under control is to eat foods that are low on the glycemic index…."

In the quote above it states that Barry Sears is a medical doctor but actually Dr. Sears is a Ph.D. Dr. Perricone recognizes sugar's toxic effects. He discusses a process known as glycation when sugar attaches to proteins and become cross-linked resulting in sagging and inflexible skin (page 74). He states on page 72 of his book that the 'real answer is to eat less sugar,' and recommends his 'anti-inflammatory diet.' He also discusses on page 105 how sugar interacts with collagen in a process known as glycosylation and says "you're much better off….dropping the added sugar from your diet."

Sugar Busters! by H. Leighton Steward, Morrison C. Bethea, M.D., Samuel S. Andrews, M.D., and Luis A. Balart, M.D. state on page 17 that **"SUGAR IS TOXIC!."**[10] Three of the authors are medical doctors and recommend a low-sugar diet, avoiding carbohydrate with a high glycemic index. It cannot be overstated or emphasized enough that what these doctors have said about the toxicity of sugar.

Michael R. Eades, M.D. and Mary Dan Eades, M.D. who have written several books on nutrition write in their popular book, *Protein Power*, that eating a high protein diet is medically and nutritionally healthier than eating the traditional 60% carbohydrate diet. They point out that the 'major diseases of Western civilization—obesity, high blood pressure, heart disease, elevated blood fats, and diabetes—have a common bond….these 'diseases' aren't diseases at all, they're symptoms of a more basic single disorder, hyperinsulinemia (excess insulin) and insulin resistance…." (*Protein Power*, p.328) They recommend controlling starches and sugars and eating a high protein diet.

Robert C. Atkins, M.D., has also written a diet advocating a high protein diet, which is similar to the *Rosacea Diet* recommending 20 grams of carbohydrate a day. Later you increase your carbohydrate until you reach a certain level. His diet is to lose weight and it works. You may read his books to confirm a diet high in protein is healthy even though other 'medical authorities' say otherwise. Here is another example of a medical doctor who still is legally practicing medicine advocating a high protein diet. I personally use his 'Carbohydrate Gram Counter' book.[11]

This should be enough evidence to convince you that I am not alone in recommending a high protein diet, avoiding sugar, drinking lots of water and taking vitamin supplements. There are medical doctors out

10. *Sugar Busters!* by H. Leighton Steward, Dr. Morrison C. Bethea, Dr. Samuel S. Andrews, and Dr. Luis A Balart, 1995, *Sugar Busters!*, LLC, page 17

11. *Dr. Atkins' New Carbohydrate Gram Counter* by Robert C. Atkins, 1996, M.D., M. Evans and Company, Inc
you can find this book listed at this url:
http://rosaceadiet.com/html/dietbooks.html
All carbohydrate gram figures used in the *Rosacea Diet* are from the above source

there and other reputable sources saying the same thing, maybe not for rosacea, but at the very least for better health. They are few, but the list is growing.

Now if your dermatologist told his patients to avoid sugar, he would get similar results as the dentist since most patients with rosacea will continue to eat as much sugar as always, and return for more prescriptions, IPL [i.e., PhotoDerm ®], Laser, ETS, nitric oxide inhibitors, and a host of treatments. This is the sad fact, that due to sugar's addictive qualities most rosaceans will not quit sugar or alter their diet. And you just might be a rosacean who will not avoid sugar or change your eating and drinking habits even after purchasing this book! You may discover the *Rosacea Diet* is too difficult for you and will not stop eating sugar or a carbohydrate diet for thirty days to even find out if it works for you! And you won't be the first. That's because most people who are on a sugar diet along with high carbohydrate have a difficult time changing their eating and drinking habits. Do you have the will power to try it? You can't give this diet thirty days of your life?

But you may say, 'I already know how sugar is bad for you, and I already avoid it in my diet, yet I STILL have rosacea!' You are to be commended, but you are a minority. Most rosaceans eat tons of sugar yet you discovered how sugar isn't healthy for you and obviously still have rosacea. Why do you have rosacea even though you avoid sugar? Have you really reduced natural sugar in your diet and a diet high in fruits and carbohydrate? What about honey or maple syrup? Are you still consuming either or both? The *Rosacea Diet* is a thirty-day diet high in protein to prove to you that you can control your rosacea. The question is, will you reduce your diet to less than 30 grams of carbohydrate a day to find out if this works for you? Most people do not know that **sugar is not good for your health**. You at least have that going for you, but you will have to follow this diet for thirty days to find out if a high protein diet controls your rosacea. So you came this far, why not try it? It is only thirty days of your life. Can't you sacrifice your eating and drinking habits for thirty days for your face? What about the majority of rosacea sufferers who eat sugar high in diet every day? Will rosaceans who eat and drink sugar decide to try this diet for thirty days? This is no picnic.

Avoiding refined sugar [sucrose] is very difficult, yet can be reduced to an extent to control rosacea symptoms. I have experimented with this over and over, having rosacea flare-ups every time I increase sucrose or natural sugar consumption. Refined sugar [sucrose] in crystallized form is artificial usually made from either sugar beets or sugarcane. Some may claim that sugar is natural, but would you call the crystallized powder heroin derived from morphine 'natural,' because it is made from the opium of a poppy? Refined table sugar doesn't occur naturally, it is an artificially manufactured process. And you may have no idea how the processed food industry has adulterated most of the food and drink you are consuming with sucrose or some other type sugar, so much so, that the typical American eats 149 pounds of it a year.[12] And the typical American diet is being promoted all over the world to eat and as a result sugar is being consumed in greater quantities each year worldwide and so is diabetes and heart disease, yet the medical authorities state that sugar in moderation is harmless.[13] And if it wasn't for people like Ralph Nador you wouldn't see the sugar content on the label of the food and drink you buy in the U.S.A. For example, even the sucrose contained in one teaspoon of catsup on my French fries usually causes my nose to break out with rosacea, not to mention the starch (which is another form of sugar) in the French Fries! One teaspoon of Catsup has 3.8 grams of carbohydrate, mostly sugar! Ten French Fries has 18 grams of carbohydrate, mostly starch (a sugar). That is just one example of sugar in your diet. What all this sugar and a diet high in carbohydrate, particularly processed food, has done to your health is manifesting as rosacea and other diseases.

---

12. See footnote 10 in this chapter

If you stop eating sugar, it may not help the cavity already formed in your tooth, but it will help prevent other cavities from forming. Does that mean you will not ever get a cavity again if you never eat sugar again? Well, no, you might get one, but your chances are drastically reduced to practically zero. Most dentists will tell you that as long as you brush your teeth and avoid sugar you will reduce your cavity possibilities to near zero in a normal healthy adult. Have you noticed how many people are losing their teeth and how much sugar they consume? Dentists know the connection sugar has with rotten teeth. They are only glad to replace your teeth with artificial ones. Do you really think that cavities are the only thing 'rotten' in your body from all the sugar you have been eating over your lifetime? And is obesity the only health problem aggravated by sugar?

So, avoiding sugar does not cure rosacea, but it definitely controls the triggers if you will avoid it for thirty days. And your overall health will improve as a result of avoiding sugar. User feedback over the past several years confirm that many *Rosacea Diet* Users experience weight loss

---

13.   **For an example of the medical profession giving their blessing on eating sugar**, notice the second most frequently asked question on the **American Diabetes Association** list:
"**2. Can I eat foods with sugar in them?**
For almost every person with diabetes, the answer is yes! Eating a piece of cake made with sugar will raise your blood glucose level. So will eating corn on the cob, a tomato sandwich, or lima beans. The truth is that sugar has gotten a bad reputation. People with diabetes can and do eat sugar. In your body, it becomes glucose, but so do the other foods mentioned above. With sugary foods, the rule is moderation. Eat too much, and 1) you'll send your blood glucose level up higher than you expected; 2) you'll fill up but without the nutrients that come with vegetables and grains; and 3) you'll gain weight. So, don't pass up a slice of birthday cake. Instead, at the next meal, eat a little less bread or potato and be sure to take a brisk walk to burn some calories."
source > http://www.diabetes.org/nutrition/faqs.asp#SugarFoods

and feel healthier with this diet. Avoiding sugar and a high carbohydrate diet probably is not good news for you but neither is rosacea.

It is now your choice, to decide whether this is true, that sugar is the catalyst that triggers rosacea and avoid it, or to continue with your status quo sugar diet including all the carbohydrate you eat and rosacea flare-ups along with whatever treatment you prefer to control your rosacea. You can control your rosacea through treatments offered by physicians or apply some alternative treatment and keep eating and drinking like you always have. Or you can try the *Rosacea Diet* just for thirty days and see if it controls your rosacea. It is only thirty days of your life.

If you are athletic and in good shape you probably eat a significant number of grams of carbohydrate for energy. You may experience fatigue and other problems if you switch to a high protein diet for thirty days. You have to weigh the balance of controlling your rosacea for thirty days with your athletic energy requirements. One suggestion is pick a time period of thirty days that you are not required to use a lot of energy which might require a sacrifice on your part. Another suggestion is ask how other *Rosacea Diet* users who are athletic have modified the *Rosacea Diet* for their lifestyle by joining the Rosacea Diet Users Support Group. Users have commented on this before and their comments are posted on the world wide web for you to read. More on this group is in a future chapter.

Even if you are not athletic, you may experience the same thing when you change your diet from a high carbohydrate diet to a high protein diet. Some report fatigue, weakness, lethargy or head aches. However, after a period of time your body adjusts to the high protein diet and many report better health later. So be patient and stick to the diet for thirty days. Don't give up just because of these aforementioned symptoms since they usually pass in time. When you change your diet your body needs to adjust and it will.

A few rosaceans who have tried this diet are already thin and do not want to lose any weight. Don't you wish you were one of them without the rosacea? If you are, this subject has come up more than a few times in the *Rosacea Diet* Users Support Group [RDUSG] and is where you can ask first hand users of the *Rosacea Diet* how they gain weight or maintain their present weight. I have some suggestions. One, join the group and ask what others have done. Two, eat plenty of heavy cream with protein powder during the thirty days as much as you can tolerate. Three, AFTER the thirty days eat plenty of mixed nuts. You may be able to tolerate a significant amount of mixed nuts AFTER the thirty days once your rosacea is controlled. If your rosacea returns after eating mixed nuts, you obviously ate too many. The thin members of the RDUSG are always looking for other ideas on increasing weight so you will have help.

You may not be able to take prescription medications for whatever reason so this information can help you as well. For those of you who are taking prescriptions or IPL [Intensity Pulsed Light, i.e., PhotoDerm ®] treatments, you may want to stop these treatments for whatever reason (s) you may think worthy. One reason may be the side effects of any medication or treatment.

There are always side effects to taking prescription medication, ETS, IPL [Intensity Pulsed Light Therapy] or other treatment. Just read the insert contained with the prescription medication that your pharmacist gives you to discover the possible side effects listed or ask the doctor the side effects or warnings given for ETS or IPL. This is what the medical community refers to as the benefit/risk ratio with treatment of a disease or injury. In treating rosacea with prescription medication or any treatment there are risks including any side effects and warnings you should be aware of, which you have the right to know about before taking such treatment. You have the choice to determine if the benefits outweigh the risks and take the treatment or decline. However, with this method of using the *Rosacea Diet* there is no risk. This diet is only for thirty days. However, your rosacea may be more difficult to control and require other treatment besides this diet, such as, treatment by a qualified physician or health care professional. And again, please consult your doctor or other health care practitioner before altering your diet. You must be getting used to my repetition by now.

Flushing and Trigger Factors

Flushing and trigger factors (or tripwires) usually come up whenever rosacea is discussed so we need to define the terms to set matters straight.

Flushing

Rosacea and flushing have almost become synonymous. This may have been the result of the work of Geoffrey Nase, Ph.D., a microvascular physiologist who wrote extensive research on rosacea flushing.[1] I have two polls on this subject currently running at both my rosaceans group and the Rosacea Diet Users Support Group that ask the question, *Do you think flushing is rosacea?* The results from this poll will prove interesting since the first group does not read this book while the second group supposedly has read it.

The statements below posted on the National Rosacea Society web site on 'What is Rosacea?' are examples of how these two words, flushing and rosacea, have almost become synonymous.

"…individuals with fair skin who tend to flush or blush easily are believed to be at greatest risk.…"

---

1. drnase.com

"Facial redness from rosacea may appear similar to a blush or sunburn, and may be caused by flushing—when a large amount of blood flows through vessels quickly and the vessels expand under the skin to handle the flow." Source > http://rosacea.org/patients/whatis.html

Dr Nase has a chapter entitled, "*Facial Flushing is the First Symptom & Primary Cause of Rosacea.*"[2] Under the subheading, *Facial Flushing is the Heart of Rosacea*, Dr. Nase wrote in bold type; "**Rosacea is caused by frequent facial flushing**."[3]

Dr. Nase states in his definition of rosacea, "…at the most basic level, rosacea is a disorder of the facial blood vessels. This disorder results in hyper-responsive blood vessels that dilate to numerous internal and external stimuli. This causes frequent facial flushing and skin changes such as facial redness, inflammatory papules, pustules, burning sensations and rhinophyma…." [source > http://drnase.com/faq.htm]

Dr. Nase defines flushing as, "In all simplicity, flushing is the result of increased blood flow through <u>dilated facial</u> blood vessels."[4]

Flushing according to my dictionary is (1) to blush, (2) to flow and spread suddenly and freely and (3) to glow suddenly red. Many rosaceans worry about factors that cause flushing so we have the NRS 'official' tripwire list[5] and Dr. Nase's 'Nine Main Triggers For Facial Flushing and Rosacea Progression.'[6] However, a blush is not rosacea. Not all flushes produce rosacea. Yes, a flush can aggravate your rosacea and you may be rightly concerned about flushing, nevertheless, a flush

---

2. *Beating Rosacea Vascular, Ocular & Acne Forms, A Must-Have Guide to Understanding & Treating Rosacea*, Geoffrey Nase, Ph.D., Nase Publications, 2001, page 49
3. ibid., page 284
4. ibid., page 285
5. http://rosacea.org/patients/materials/tripwires.html

is not rosacea. People who do not have rosacea flush and there are rosaceans who flush and not experience a rosacea flare-up.

My point is not to confuse flushing with rosacea. Flushing may be a concern, but it does not have to be an obsession with rosaceans. Dr. Nase's definition quoted above[7] says the 'disorder' causes 'frequent facial flushing,' not the flushing causes the rosacea. The National Rosacea Society says the 'facial redness from rosacea MAY be caused by flushing,' not *is* caused by flushing. Even Dr. Nase points out in answer to the question, 'Why does the...flushing...advance into the...more severe stages?' by answering,

> "Although the exact cellular reasons are not yet fully understood, vascular specialists believe that rosacea progressively worsens due to vascular changes that take place in areas of frequent flushing."[8]

Trigger Factors

The NRS does not distinguish tripwires from trigger factors using both terms to mean the same thing, which can be anything that MAY produce a rosacea flare-up.[9]

The booklet, *Coping With Rosacea*, National Rosacea Society, page 1 states:

---

6. See footnote 2 above, page 285, Dr. Nase lists the **Nine Main Triggers for Facial Flushing and Rosacea Progression** as follows: (1) Nerves (2) Skin Irritation (3) Sun (4) Environmental Factors (Heat, Cold, & Wind) (5) Topical Steroids (6) Stress (Neural & Hormonal) (7) Food & Beverage (8) Immune system (9) Free Radicals
7. http://drnase.com/faq.htm
8. See footnote 2, this chapter, page 285, also page 51 under the subheading, *Why Does Facial Flushing Get Worse Over Time?*
9. *Coping With Rosacea*, National Rosacea Society, page 1

"…Rosacea tripwires are factors that may cause a rosacea sufferer to experience a flare-up—a more intense outbreak of redness, bumps or pimples. While the list of potential tripwires ranges from weather to emotions to foods, nearly all are related to flushing.
As a rule, anything that causes a rosacea sufferer to flush may trigger a flare-up…."

Rosacea is better defined not in terms of flushing but instead as "chronic, relapsing and potentially life-disruptive disorder of the facial skin" Source > http://rosacea.org/patients/whatis.html

Sometimes rosacea is referred to as 'adult acne' which is not a bad definition. Flushing or trigger factors may be getting more of the limelight but rosacea is the stop light. Making a list of potential flush factors may be helpful but they are not set in stone. There is no list of proven rosacea trigger factors that in every rosacean produces a rosacea flare-up. In fact there is no proven single flushing factor that in every case produces a rosacea flare-up in every rosacean! Any flushing rosacea trigger factor or tripwire only MAY produce a rosacea flare-up, no matter who makes up the list.

Dr. Nase says on page 288 of his book "Rosacea is caused by a combination of factors…due to cumulative insults from several different triggers." As you can see from this, who really knows what is triggering your flushing, much less anyone's rosacea? I suppose if we all had the time and money we could hire some specialist (hopefully a dermatologist) who could figure all this out for us but do you have the money or the time? We are all in the same boat trying to figure what is triggering our rosacea. This book centers on diet triggers. However, when you bring in all the other tripwires/triggers into this equation you get a complicated mathematical possibility with rosacea triggers. While you are eating and drinking there is a host of other issues you may be dealing with that loads a plethora of triggers for your rosacea. Can you positively rule the other trigger factors out when you are eating and drinking? Then you are one smart cookie.

The reason I bring this up is that the National Rosacea Society has the 'official' trigger (tripwire) factor list that includes diet triggers that usually relates somehow to flushing.

Dr. Nase's nine-trigger list all relates to flushing. I repeatedly keep getting questions from users of the *Rosacea Diet* why the foods I recommend to eat are on the NRS list to avoid. I wrote this chapter to explain the quandary of trigger factors and flushing. No one has ever written a trigger list that is bulletproof. All the lists have holes in it since you may not 'trigger' your rosacea from one of the bullets on the list. One day the NRS may list sugar and high carbohydrate as a trigger factor and then it will be 'official,' and until that time please reread this chapter. The NRS does not recognize sugar's inflammatory properties or list sugar as a trigger. Nor does the NRS list 'free radicals' as a trigger factor but Dr. Nase does when he lists his nine major rosacea trigger factors[10]. Remember that a food or drink on any 'official' list as a trigger factor or tripwire may NOT produce a rosacea flare-up.

---

10.   See footnote number 6, this chapter

Protein and Fat
—Essential for Life!

Essential food and drink may be obvious to you but you may be surprised at the following statement. Protein, fat, and water are essential to life, but carbohydrate is not. If you were on a desert island or the moon you can survive on protein, fat and water. If you strictly only had carbohydrate you would eventually die. Why?

Carbohydrate is a word derived from Greek meaning 'carbon plus water.' All carbohydrate is composed of units of sugars and could be called the *dessert* of food. Carbohydrate is broken down to glucose, which is essential to human life. Glucose and oxygen is essential for cell survival and the fuel of the body. However, you can obtain glucose from protein and fat. You cannot get protein or fat from carbohydrate. It is impossible and an indisputable fact. You can obtain glucose from all three food groups, carbohydrate, protein and fat. But on a desert island if you only had carbohydrate you would die! For example, if the only food source was table sugar, a carbohydrate, and you even had water, eventually you would actually go bonkers and die.[1] You would

---

1. *Sugar Blues*, William Dufty, 1975, Warner Books, Inc., describes in the chapter, *Dead Dogs and Englishman*, about a shipwrecked vessel in 1793 with five surviving sailors marooned for just nine days rescued in a wasted condition due to starvation. The sailors had subsisted on a diet of sugar and rum. As Dufty wrote on page 137, "Refined sugar is lethal when ingested by humans because it provides only that which nutritionists describe as empty or naked calories. In addition, sugar is worse than nothing because it drains and leeches the body of precious vitamins and minerals through the demand its digestion, detoxification, and elimination make upon one's entire system."

die of malnutrition. You need protein and fat. Of course you also need certain vitamins, minerals, fiber, and a host of other things to survive, but I am trying to make a point about carbohydrate. Try to be open-minded and give me a break. My purpose in this chapter is to establish protein and fat as essential to life. I am on a roll here and you need to keep up.

Most plants (vegetables, grains, fruits, nuts, etc.) contain mostly carbohydrate but may contain also some protein and fat. So when you eat plants you may obtain all three-food groups. Fish, seafood, eggs, and meat contain protein and fat but usually no carbohydrate and in rare exceptions have trace amounts of carbohydrate. A three-ounce slice of beef liver, for instance, contains 22.4 grams of protein, 9 grams of fat, and 4.5 grams of carbohydrate. Who would ever think that liver has carbohydrate! Dairy may have all three-food groups but in some cases zero carbohydrate. Cream has fat and protein but no carbohydrate!

The human health requirement for protein established by most reputable health authorities is between 50 to 100 grams a day depending on several factors such as age, weight, sex, activity, etc. If you are in a concentration camp the above requirement for protein will keep you alive, but probably not very healthy. You obviously need more than 50 to 100 grams of protein! But remember that if you fail to get protein you will die. If you don't get ENOUGH protein you will be unhealthy. Absolute fact. There is a debate among health professionals that you can eat too much protein. However this debate is foolish when you simply think of the Eskimo who at one time lived on a diet high in protein and fat, and some Eskimo may still eat this way! But the sad fact is that more and more Eskimo are drinking soft drinks and eating twinkies. At one time carbohydrate was simply rarely available to the Eskimo, yet this group survived on a high protein/fat diet.

Think about overeating protein. Imagine the Eskimo overeating protein. Will the Eskimo die or be unhealthy? Are you going to tell the Eskimo to stop eating a high protein diet? Imagine a *diet authority* browbeating the high protein/fat diet of the Eskimo or claiming that what the Eskimo ate is unhealthy or that he may have a disease creating a problem digesting protein? But these same health critics on diets will browbeat any high protein diet and site all sorts of reasons, shouting about the waste products created in high protein diets. These pale into insignificance when you mention the Eskimo. How did the Eskimo manage the waste products from eating a high protein diet and survive for all these millenniums? For that matter the Australian aborigine is another group to bring up. There are other groups or cultures eating a high protein, high fat diet and survived.

Lets discuss the usual warnings given for eating a high protein diet. People with certain diseases have problems processing protein, like gout, and so *diet authorities* browbeat high protein diets based on the possibility that a person might have a disease that impairs digesting protein, so therefore, according to this logic high protein diets are bad. Actually this is begging the question. The issue is whether eating a high protein diet is unhealthy, not whether a person has a problem digesting protein. The critics of high protein diets say eating a high protein diet may result in not being able to digest protein, which has never been proven. It is just a theory. Reasonably most people do not have diseases that would create a problem digesting protein and can eat as much protein as they want. The other issue is with waste products produced from eating a high protein diet that may produce health problems. Again, this is begging the question. The issue is whether eating a high protein diet is healthy, not the possibility of having a problem removing waste from a high protein diet. Most humans have no problem handling waste products from protein and there is no evidence that humans eating a high protein diet can not handle the waste products in the normal manner. The waste products from protein are simply eliminated from the body in the normal manner. Drs. Eades of *Protein Power* fame have explained in their books that eating a high protein diet is healthy and they are not the only medical doctors saying this. High protein diets are healthy even though the health critics lambaste those who endorse such diets. Remember the Eskimo.

Fat is required for human health and the health authorities have established the magic number of no more than thirty percent of your total daily calories[2] should be fat. On the Greek Island of Crete the traditional diet constitutes 40 percent fat of the total caloric intake. The rate of heart disease on this island is less than on the island of Japan, where the traditional diet is only 8 to 10 per cent fat. Imagine the *diet authorities* warning the inhabitants of Crete for eating too much fat! Sounds like a great place to live and eat. We should all check out what the Cretans eat.

Thirty percent of a 2,000-calorie diet would amount to 600 calories or 66.7 grams of fat. Fat has nine calories per gram. Fat is what nutritionists and health authorities call lipids. All lipids are divided into three groups, triglycerides, phospholipids, and sterols. All three are essential to life. If you are on that desert island you must obtain all three forms of fat or you die. That is a fact. The triglycerides are the fat composed of three essential fatty acids floating around in your blood that can be burned by the body cells for energy if needed. That is just one thing triglycerides are good for. If you don't have glucose in your blood, triglycerides may be used to burn energy by converting fatty acids into glucose. Amazing, isn't it? And you thought triglycerides are bad, didn't you? Who told you that? You need triglycerides. You may be worrying about your triglyceride level in your blood because your doctor told

---

2. "The 30 percent limit on fat was essentially drawn from thin air."—*Scientific American*, January 2003, Rebuilding the Food Guide Pyramid, Walter C. Willett and Meir J. Stampfer

you to worry about it. But you better be happy you have triglyerides in your body because you need them.

Fat is used in your cells as a membrane. Myelin, the fatty material that sheathes nerve cells, is composed of fat. These are just some examples of how you need fat. Can you eat too much fat and have problems? That is an unctuous subject. Think again of the Eskimo. How did the Eskimo survive on a diet high in fat and protein? They did it despite all the health warnings from the *diet authorities* that eating too much fat is unhealthy. The Australian aborigines in times past or present also ate a high fat/protein diet in the bush. Imagine the *diet authorities* criticizing their diet?

Fat is probably the most studied and talked about food of *diet authorities* and nutritionists. The alleged dangers of fat are notorious and swollen. Don't you just love puns? You can read all about saturated, unsaturated, monounsaturated, polyunsaturated, cholesterol, lipoproteins (HDLs and LDLs), triglycerides, etc., and get insulated in a fat discussion with your health care provider who no doubt has some very entrenched beliefs about fat. Just about everyone puts trans fats down which is no doubt a good idea. Just remember that all health authorities recommend you eat no more than 66.7 grams of fat or the magic number of thirty percent of your total caloric intake. Another big debate is that the red meat contains 'bad' fat while the 'good' fat is in plants, fish, and seafood. Stop and think of the American Indian who ate a diet high in the red meat of the buffalo and other game animals. Can you imagine a nutritionist putting down an American Indian eating all that fat from red meat?

It is universal that you can eat fat since just about every *diet authority* allows up to the magic number 30 per cent of the total caloric intake. The debate is over which fats and if you eat more than thirty per cent. But you can eat fat, which is my point! Fat is not the bad guy. We need fat, and fat is good! Fat really is the good guy! The mantra from the health authorities for the past thirty or more years that 'fat is bad' is no doubt deeply rooted in your heart. But take heart, you need fat! Start repeating over and over 'fat is good, fat is good.' You need fat for human survival.

Everyone needs cholesterol to survive which is fat. Cholesterol is in your cells, your organs, and glands. Cholesterol is essential for human health. It is used as the base for building steroid hormones such as estrogen and testosterone. Bile is made from cholesterol. We need cholesterol. Why has cholesterol been given such a bad reputation? There are many reasons but it isn't because you do not need cholesterol since you do. If you are on that desert island you must somehow obtain cholesterol or you die. You may have a problem with cholesterol but it is not because you don't need cholesterol! If you don't have cholesterol you die! I am repeating this because the health authorities have given cholesterol such a bad reputation that you may feel that your cholesterol level somehow is related to being a friend of Hitler. Your cholesterol level can bring you into some sort of panic attack because of all this worry over what it should be. Rosaceans don't need any more stress so stop worrying about your cholesterol level during the thirty days of this diet. You can go back and worry all you want after the thirty days are over and your rosacea is controlled. Then ask you dermatologist about your cholesterol level after you have eaten a high protein diet and see what he says happened to your cholesterol level in thirty days. The results may surprise you. Cholesterol is essential fat. So give cholesterol and fat a break. You deserve to eat your fat or your cholesterol without guilt and you can eat up to thirty per cent of fat in your diet!

Now one of the big debates is over the 'bad' cholesterol and sorting out the 'good' cholesterol. The 'bad' cholesterol is actually a misnomer since both are essential for human health. Again it is the amount and ratios that are debated and whether your high and low density lipoproteins are within the norms. But there is no debate over the fact that we need both types of high and low density lipoproteins. Actually you have been mislead by the *diet authorities* because in your mind the HDLs and LDLs are fat, but as the acronym points out they are protein particles carrying cholesterol. Technically they are protein carrying fat, hence, *lipoprotein*. They are the same particle depending on whether the particle takes cholesterol into the blood vessels (LDLs) or carries it out of the body (HDLs). So much for your cholesterol lesson. Anyway, we need both for survival. 30 per cent fat is ok. 'Fat is good' should be your new mantra. Cholesterol is good too! Three cheers for triglycerides!!!

Now the final food group is carbohydrate. If you just had plenty of table sugar on that desert island (which is a carbohydrate) and plenty of water you would still die of malnutrition if that is all you had. The human health requirement for carbohydrate is zero.[3] That is a fact. *Diet authorities* have recommended a diet high in carbohydrate over the last century especially since 1992 when the USDA officially endorsed carbohydrate, a food group not essential for human health. Americans have high carbohydrated their life style ever since. Health and *diet authorities* have praised the carbohydrate to the maximum, a food group not essential for survival, and instead attacked fat, giving minimal praise to protein. In the minds of the typical American, the health authorities have established the mantra 'fat is bad' and 'carbohydrate are good.' Protein is minimized with barely an honorable mention giving you the idea that if you eat too much protein you will eat too much fat and you should worry about this.

However, a growing group of *diet authorities* have bravely published that a diet high in protein is healthy. This book joins the force against

3.   *Protein Power* by Michael R. Eades, M.D. and Mary Dan Eades, M.D., 16, Bantam Books, page 8, footnote at bottom

carbohydrate proponents. Eating a high carbohydrate diet is not healthy. The results of obesity and other health problems of Americans eating a high carbohydrate diet over the past century is evidence that it doesn't work. You need protein and fat. You don't need carbohydrate. That does not mean you have to completely avoid carbohydrate. You just need to minimize carbohydrate in your diet. What carbohydrate does for food is add sugar and we all like the taste of sugar. Carbohydrate is simply different units of sugar that is the dessert of the three food groups. However, you should be eating a low carbohydrate diet to control your rosacea, lose weight and feel healthy. And since you can live without carbohydrate, minimizing them for thirty days poses no health risks. You will control your rosacea. Other health problems may improve. And you will lose weight. You will feel healthier. And if you try the *Rosacea Diet* for thirty days which is an extreme low carbohydrate diet for thirty days you will find that you rosacea is controlled or minimized. After the thirty days you can eat whatever you want, but I suggest eat low carbohydrate and instead change to a high protein diet lifestyle and eat no more than thirty percent fat!

Protein can be converted to glucose, which is essential for human life and you can obtain glucose from protein through gluconeogenesis, which is the subject of the another chapter.

If you are athletic and in good shape you probably eat a significant number of grams of carbohydrate for energy. You may experience fatigue and other problems if you switch to a high protein diet for thirty days. So try to pick a thirty day period when you can adjust your metabolism to a high protein diet without undue physical stress that requires carbohydrate energy. After the thirty days you can evaluate what you learned from this to adjust your carbohydrate intake for energy. You should realize the benefit of reducing sugar's toxic effects on your body from this experience with a healthier body. Many of the 'energy bars' are loaded with sugar, whether it is sucrose or some other type sugar. Avoid them like the plague. Protein bars can contain more than 25 to 30 grams of carbohydrate. Avoid them too. Find protein bars with minimal or zero carbohydrate and no sugar substitutes.

Even if you are not athletic, you may experience the same thing when you change your diet from a high carbohydrate diet to a high protein diet. Some report fatigue, weakness, lethargy, or head aches. However, after a period of time your body adjusts to the high protein diet and many report better health later. Your metabolism is changing. So be patient and stick to the diet for thirty days. Don't give up just because of these aforementioned symptoms since they usually pass in time. When you change your diet your body needs to adjust and it will.

Rosacea Diet is a high protein diet for thirty days and is limited to 30 grams of carbohydrate a day. After the thirty days you can return to your high carbohydrate diet or eat all the sugar or sugar substitutes you want. What is the point of doing this for thirty days? To prove to yourself that you will control your rosacea, lose weight or feel healthier. Sugar in your diet is not good for you. High carbohydrate must be avoided for thirty days to change your metabolism to prove this. It takes thirty days to see any significant results. When you go back to the way your were eating before changing to *Rosacea Diet* your weight or your health problems return. Eating the *Rosacea Diet* works. It is only thirty days of your life. I can't convince you. You must convince yourself and the only way is to try the *Rosacea Diet*.

Some complain also of constipation when changing over from a high carbohydrate diet to a high protein diet. Your metabolism is changing. You currently have an insulin dominant metabolism. To help eliminate constipation the number one solution is to drink plenty of water. Just water. Lots of water. More than you have ever drunk before. Water. Drinking large volumes of water for thirty days usually poses no health risks but I have a chapter on water you should read before you begin this diet. Also read suggestion number four in the chapter, *Ten Suggestions for the Thirty-Day Diet Plan*, about water. Ten twelve-ounce glasses of water should be enough water if you are having problems with constipation. Second, increase the magnesium supplement to double or triple the suggested amount in the chapter *Vitamins and Supplements*. Third, increase the fish oil supplement to double or triple in the same chapter. Fourth, you need more fiber. Use Oat Bran or Flaxseed bran. A half-ounce of oat bran has 7.5 grams of carbohydrate. You can also get fiber from cabbage or other green vegetable. The next chapter deals with fiber and *effective* carbohydrate and how to deduct the fiber from the carbohydrate total.

Some may be concerned with the hormones, antibiotics and other possible contaminates in the meat. Others may be concerned with the PCBs, mercury and other contaminates in fish, particularly salmon. If you have issues with this, no doubt, you are rightly concerned. Finding meat or fish without contaminates is possible if you can afford it. The demand for uncontaminated meat and fish will increase without a doubt.

Fiber and Effective Carbohydrate

When you read the Nutrition Facts Label (see the chapter *Nutrition Facts Label*) under Carbohydrate it lists *Fiber*. Dietary fiber is not a source of energy for humans because we cannot break the bonds that hold fiber's sugar units together because we don't have the enzymes to do it. Cows do, but humans can't. Therefore, fiber adds no calories to your diet and cannot be converted to glucose. Hence when you read the Nutrition Facts Label you may deduct the fiber content from the total Carbohydrate Gram content. Many food labels do this for you since this is the cool thing to do if you are counting carbohydrate. Sugar Alcohol sometimes is also deducted from the total carbohydrate content on these products and this is stated on the label. Labeling on a product sometimes states that the total **EFFECTIVE CARBOHY-DRATE** is less than the total amount in the Nutrition Facts Label. What should a rosacean do with this?

Many products do not state the *effective carbohydrate*. If a product does not state this, you may deduct the *fiber* from the total carbohydrate content. The Nutrition Facts Label is set up this way. Note the *Fiber* in the total and deduct it. This is how you have the *effective carbohydrate*.

During the thirty days of the *Rosacea Diet* I have specifically said NOT to consume any sugar alcohol (see the chapter *Sugars to Avoid*). So please do this. AFTER the thirty days you can experiment all you want with sugar alcohol. This is to assure that your rosacea will be controlled. You can't control your rosacea until you rule out sugar alcohol.

If your rosacea is controlled by avoiding sugar alcohol for thirty days and then you consume sugar alcohol and your rosacea breaks out, what do you conclude? Now back to fiber.

Dr. Nase sent me this interesting email about fiber:

From: "Dr. Geoffrey Nase"
Date: Fri, 08 Aug 2003

Brady,

We are finding out that dietary fiber intake with a meal substantially slows down simple sugar absorption, amino acid absorption and overall nutrient absorption. This is partly due to binding factors, actions on the lipophilic/cotransport systems through the intestinal wall and other yet undefined mechanisms. This helps to decrease glucose spikes (especially in diabetics) and the postprandial peripheral vasodilation elicited to deliver the nutrients to organs such as the skin. Citrucel and vegetable based fibers do help to decrease skin flushing in a significant number of rosacea sufferers. Experimentation is needed though to find the right concentration and the timing (taking it 30 minutes prior to meal vs. during meal). It is interesting to speculate that these new carbohydrate binder pills may also have similar actions. This does help a significant number. Hope this helps some.

Dietary fibre, physicochemical properties and their relationship to health.
Blackwood AD, Salter J, Dettmar PW, Chaplin MF.
Food Research Centre, South Bank University,103 Borough Road, London SE1 0AA, England.

Dietary carbohydrate that escape digestion and absorption in the small intestine include non-digestible oligosaccharides (carbohydrate with a degree of polymerisation between three and ten), resistant starch and non-starch polysaccharides. The physiological effects of this heterogeneous mixture of substrates are partly predictable on the basis of their physico-chemical properties. Monosaccharide composition and chain conformation influence the rate and extent of fermentation. Water-holding capacity affects stool weight and intestinal transit time. Viscous polysaccharides can cause delayed gastric emptying and slower transit through the small bowel, resulting in the reduced rate of nutrient absorption. Polysaccharides with large hydrophobic surface areas have potentially important roles in the binding of bile acids, carcinogens and mutagens. Ispaghula is capable of binding bile acids through a large number of weak binding sites on the polysaccharide structure, and having greatest effect on the potentially more harmful secondary bile acids deoxycholic acid and lithocholic acid.

Unabsorbable carbohydrate and diabetes: Decreased post-prandial hyperglycaemia.
Jenkins DJ, Goff DV,LeedsAR, Alberti KG, Wolever TM, Gassull MA, Hockaday TD.

Two test meals were taken in random order on separate days by 8 non-insulin-requiring diabetic volunteers after 14-hour overnight fasts. Addition of 16 g guar and 10 g pectin to the control meal containing 106 g carbohydrate decreased markedly and significantly the rise in blood-glucose between 30 and 90 minutes and also resulted in significantly lower insulin levels between 30 and 120 minutes. When these meals were fed to 3 insulin-dependent diabetic subjects, a similar flattening of the post-prandial glucose rise ensued. This addition of certain forms of dietary fibre to the diet of diabetics significantly decreases post-prandial hyperglycaemia and would be expected to improve the control of blood-glucose concentration.

Publication Types:
Clinical Trial—Controlled Trial

Fiber and diabetes.
Anderson JW, Midgley WR, Wedman B.

Plant fibers have important influences on gastrointestinal physiology and the absorption of many nutrients. Certain fibers delay the absorption of carbohydrate and result in less postprandial hyperglycemia. Because the intake of plant fibers lowers plasma glucose concentrations and decreases glycosuria, high-fiber foods may be useful in the management of diabetes mellitus. Consumption of selected fibers and fiber-rich foods lowers serum cholesterol values and may lower triglyceride concentrations. Plant fiber intake may lead to mineral depletion or vitamin deficiency, but this has not been observed in several long-term studies. Further work is required to delineate the therapeutic utility of plant fibers in the diet of persons with diabetes and to assess the undesirable effects of fiber intake. In our opinion, persons with diabetes who are eating very low-fiber diets would benefit from an increase in plant fiber intake from whole grains, legumes, and vegetables.

Geoffrey
======================
Dr. Geoffrey Nase

Ph.D. Microvascular Physiologist
www.drnase.com

This no doubt gives you food for thought on fiber and effective carbo-hydrate. You may increase the fiber in you diet and according to all the evidence you can deduct this from your carbohydrate intake. This is good news for rosaceans. Thanks to Dr. Nase for this insight I have added this chapter.

Protein Synthesis and Gluconeogenesis

Many do not know what happens to the proteins you eat or the fact that you can get glucose from protein. Proteins are made up of carbon, hydrogen, and oxygen atoms combined into certain amino acids containing nitrogen. There are 22 different amino acids that your body needs, nine are essential, which means you cannot synthesize them in your body and therefore you obtain them from food. The other thirteen amino acids your body needs, the nonessential ones can be obtained from the food you eat or you can manufacture them yourself from fats, carbohydrate, and other amino acids. Basically your body uses proteins to build new cells, maintain tissues, and synthesize new proteins. Proteins from foods are broken down into their component amino acids by digestive enzymes (specialized proteins), while other enzymes inside your body cells synthesize new proteins by reassembling amino acids into specific compounds that your body needs. This process is called *protein synthesis*. About half the dietary protein you consume each day goes to make enzymes, many of which have to do with digesting food using certain vitamins and minerals for this task. New cells need protein. Nucleoproteins are chemicals in the nucleus of every living cell made up of amino acids and nucleic acids. The carbon, hydrogen, and oxygen left over after *protein synthesis* is complete is converted to glucose and used for energy. The nitrogen left over is converted to urea, most of which is excreted in urine. What *protein synthesis* does for you is wonderful since you can obtain glucose from protein that is essential for life since your cells need glucose and oxygen. You may have thought that you need glucose from carbohydrate, but the **actual amount of carbohydrate required by humans for health is zero** (see footnote 3, page 50 and the chapter *Protein and Fat Essential for Life*). You can obtain glucose from protein through *gluconeogenesis* when amino acids are converted into glucose by the liver from non-carbohydrate food sources like protein.

Protein synthesis and gluconeogenesis effect body metabolism. This process is dependent on the liver, pancreas and other organs being in balance. What we eat can affect these organs in the way they function as a whole. If you are changing from a 60% or higher carbohydrate diet your metabolism takes time to change, possibly weeks, to release glucagon into your bloodstream and to jump-start gluconeogensis. And in time, usually about thirty days your body metabolism will adjust. You may notice some quirks in your body as you adjust from an insulin dominant metabolism to a glucagon dominant metabolism.

The high-quality proteins come from meat, fish, seafood, poultry, eggs and dairy products that are absorbed more efficiently without much waste to synthesize proteins. The proteins from plants often have limited amounts of some amino acids and our bodies do not absorb them as easily or use them as efficiently as animal proteins so their nutritional quality is considered a low-quality protein. The prime exception is the soybean, which is packed with the nine essential amino acids and is the number one source of protein for vegetarians, which is the subject of another chapter.

A high protein diet along with protein synthesis can help you control your weight and feel healthier. *Gluconeogenesis* manufactures the glucose you need for energy. Remember that your grandmother or your mom said that you need chicken soup when you were sick? Chicken soup is protein. It heals. That is what rosaceans need, protein.

Glucagon vs. Insulin

You may have heard of insulin but you probably have not heard of glucagon. Both hormones are made by the pancreas and regulate blood sugar. Insulin, as you probably know, enables you to digest and metabolize glucose from carbohydrate, fat or protein. Your body cells cannot burn the glucose without insulin. Impossible. Insulin is essential for human survival. If you run out of insulin you are in trouble. Doctors love to prescribe prescription insulin if your pancreas can not manufacture it anymore since insulin is essential for human survival.

Glucagon is released when blood glucose is low. Glucagon metabolizes glycogen (stored glucose) first and then the fat or protein so that body cells obtain energy. Conversion of protein into glucose was described in the chapter, *Protein Synthesis and Gluconeogenesis*.

A diet high in carbohydrate stimulates insulin production in the blood, especially when the diet includes a generous amount of sugar. This may result over time into insulin resistance in which the receptors no longer respond properly to insulin or hyperinsulinemia, which means simply having too much insulin in the blood. Over time diabetes may result. While the medical authorities keep saying over and over that a sugar diet is not a factor in any of these conditions, any one with half a brain can come to the same conclusion as you just did. If 2 out of 3 diabetics suffer heart attacks or stroke it doesn't take a medical degree or a Ph.D. to understand that sugar is a factor in all these diseases. What has happened is simply eating a diet high in sugar over the years taxes the poor old pancreas who has been cranking out enormous amounts of insulin until it is simply worn out and cries 'Don't you get it? I am out of insulin!' Medical *and diet authorities* insist that eating sugar have nothing to do with diabetes, heart disease, stroke or cancer? The medical profession is ready to give you prescriptions and treatment for diabetes, heart disease or stroke.

Now the classic response is, 'What about all these people in their seventies or eighties or more who ate sugar all their life who are healthy?' My response is they are few and the majority is already either dead or is on their way out with diabetes, heart disease, stroke, cancer or some other disease, not evening mentioning rosacea. If you take a revolver with one bullet in the chamber of six slots, spin it and then click it to your head you have a one in six possibility that the gun will go off and kill or hurt you. Now take that gun and hand it to the next fellow and do this for millions of people over seventy or eighty years. Sure, there will be a few still alive in their seventy and eighties. But how many were shot or seriously wounded? Would you accept that gun and pull the trigger to your head? Many do when they eat sugar in such huge quantities. When you eat sugar in your diet along with a high carbohydrate diet you are wearing your pancreas out trying to make insulin. Remember that insulin is essential for human life. You need it. You only have so much to make and then, poof, no more. The *Sugar Age* began at the beginning of the eighteenth century. When humans ate food before the advent of the *Sugar age* the pancreas could handle the carbohydrate the average human ate. Before the *Sugar age* diabetes was rare. With the advent of the *Sugar Age* diabetes, heart disease, stroke, and cancer have risen in greater percentages since 1700. Sugar is a factor in these diseases without a doubt.

The pancreas releases glucagon when your blood glucose is *low*. After burning up all the glycogen, glucagon starts working on fat and protein to metabolize glucose to burn in your cells. You want to have a glucagon dominate metabolism. No doubt before the *Sugar Age* mankind's metabolism was glucagon dominate. Since the *Sugar Age* began mankind has steadily changed over from bodies that were glucagon dominant to an insulin dominant metabolism. You need to save every drop of insulin you have left. Think of this formula:

L = your life span
X = amount of insulin your pancreas can make
D = your diet

$$L = X/D$$

God only knows what your pancreas can make over a lifetime of eating all the sugar you consume along with a high carbohydrate diet. You will eventually know yourself when the doctor says you have diabetes. You think you can be one of the few who make it into the eighties eating and drinking sugar the whole way with your little 'ole pancreas pumping its little heart out squeezing the last bit of insulin it has to produce for your sugar sweet life? Go for it. Pull the trigger and you are wiping out your pancreas or at the very least increasing your chances for health problems. But what if you are not one of the few who make it into your seventies or eighties with a healthy pancreas?

And quality of life is not in the above formula until you develop diabetes, heart disease, cancer, stroke or something else. You want to try factoring that in? Treatment for these diseases is not fun and your quality of life isn't what it used to be if you get any of these diseases. And rosacea is already a part of the equation in your health. You now have to consider treatment for rosacea and all of the problems this disease has dumped on you.

If sugar is a factor in these diseases, no doubt there is a long list of other diseases in which sugar is a factor. And you don't think diabetes is serious? Think again. It is dead serious. Remember that two out of three diabetics die of heart disease or stroke. Many die of cancer. On the death certificates of these diabetics who die of heart disease, stroke or cancer do you think the cause of death is diabetes? No the certificate lists heart disease, stroke or cancer and the statistics show these as the leading cause of death. The current number of people with diabetes worldwide is 170 million in 2003. Will you be the next one added to this statistic?

When you eat a low carbohydrate diet you will need insulin to metabolize the glucose. You want it available. You shouldn't want prescription insulin that comes from a prescription. You want the real insulin made by your own pancreas. One possibility you may assure you have insulin is to have a glucagon dominant blood metabolism. Right now you probably have an insulin dominant metabolism. To change your metabolism will cost you. What will it cost? Your suffering this change with a thirty-day diet suggested in this book. The cost is well worth it. Your weight will drop and you will feel healthier. **And you will see improvement in your rosacea!** In thirty days you will have a glucagon dominate metabolism and notice the big difference in your rosacea, weight loss and health if you follow the 30-day diet plan in this book. You are the *diet authority* and can choose whether you want a glucagon dominant metabolism or let your insulin dominance remain the same and see if you make it into your seventies or eighties healthy. You can try some other way to control your rosacea. I think the odds are against those with an insulin dominant metabolism. Seriously consider insulin vs. glucagon. Glucagon should win. You are the only one who can help glucagon win.

So you immediately say, 'I am a rosacean! Why are you talking to me about diabetes and other disease?' If sugar is a factor in obesity and cavities in teeth, do you think eating a diet high in sugar is a factor in diabetes even when the medical and diet authorities say it isn't a factor? The medical and diet authorities minimize sugar toxic effects. Do you think that sugar isn't a factor in the development of rosacea? Sugar has wreaked havoc with your entire body metabolism until it has shown up on your face as rosacea. The way to control rosacea is to have a glucagon dominant metabolism. The *Rosacea Diet* will control your rosacea.

Fat vs. Sugar

Something needs to be said about concerns over sugar vs. fat. For years the medical profession and nutritionists have warned that fat is bad for your health with very little concern about sugar. You have to decide if you can stop worrying about fat for thirty days to see if the *Rosacea Diet* controls your rosacea and you feel healthier. After the thirty days, you can avoid all the fat you want especially which type of fat. Just remember that all health authorities say that you may have up to 30 percent of your total calories from fat, which amounts to 66.7 grams of fat in a 2000-calorie diet! (See the chapter *Protein and Fat—Essential for Life!*) If you take my suggestion to read *Protein Power* you will discover that the 'fat is bad' myth is just that, a myth. The *Rosacea Diet* will actually lower your 'bad' cholesterol and raise your 'good' cholesterol levels. What is bad is eating sugar, highly refined processed food, or a diet high in carbohydrate. Over the years this taxes your body's immune system or upsets your metabolism to a point of being unable to cope with diseases like rosacea, diabetes or other vascular disorders. Eating sugar in your diet is more of a concern than eating fat. Mankind has consumed sugar and refined carbohydrate in processed food in such huge quantities only for the last couple of hundred years or so when sugarcane from the West Indies began to be shipped to the rest of the world. Before this, mankind had a diet that mainly consisted of meat, fish, fowl, dairy, eggs, grains, vegetables, fruits and very little honey or maple syrup. Sweets were just not available in the amount consumed today. Sucrose in the form of a white crystal was not known for thousands of years! But for the last couple of hundred years or so, sugar consumption has grown at an astronomical rate. NEVER has mankind eaten the amount of sugar that the world consumes now. The typical

American eats 149 pounds of sugar a year! That is right, ONE HUN-DRED FORTY NINE pounds! And the *diet authorities* keep saying that heart disease and diabetes, which are vascular disorders, have little to do with sugar, and fat is the culprit? These authorities point to FAT as the problem and continue to say that SUGAR is hardly a worry. Heart disease is still the number one killer for Americans and diabetes is the tenth leading cause of death, even though the medical authorities bless low fat diets. For millenniums mankind has not had to use the pancreas to produce the amount of insulin required to eat the amount of sugar the average American eats. When sugar was not eaten in such huge quantity mankind gave little concern about eating fat. It is only in the twentieth century that the medical authorities became con-cerned over fat, with barely a concern over the sugar consumption in such huge amounts. History may show someday that the large amount of sugar consumption during the *Sugar Age* was a factor in many of the diseases resulting from an insulin dominant metabolism. So you have to decide, fat verses sugar for thirty days. Just enjoy the protein and whatever fat comes along with it. It's only thirty days. You can go back to worrying about fat after the thirty days. What you should worry about is sugar in your diet, not fat. And what if the *Rosacea Diet* really controls your rosacea and you feel healthier? The only way to know is try it for thirty days. And I urge you again to please read *Protein Power* and *Sugar Busters!* Protein is actually good for you and will help control your weight and you will feel healthier. This is what the *Rosacea Diet* is all about. When using oil, I recommend Extra Virgin Olive Oil, all natural cold pressed. Thirty-days eating a high protein diet along with whatever fat comes with it is not a health risk.

Sugar Suffice Is Not Nice

Sugar and spice and everything nice. Sugar suffice is not nice.

The above two statements cannot be both true. Mom and the processed food industry conditioned you that sugar is nice. Sugar is not nice. Sugar is toxic.

Sugar Busters! by H. Leighton Steward, Morrison C. Bethea, M.D., Samuel S. Andrews, M.D., and Luis A Balart, M.D. states on page 17 that "**SUGAR IS TOXIC!**" Three of the authors are medical doctors and recommend a low-sugar diet, avoiding carbohydrate with a high glycemic index. Do you get it? Medical doctors are saying that sugar is toxic. How can they write a book stating that sugar is toxic and still be licensed physicians? That is because it is true, sugar is toxic and is cumulative over time.

William Dufty summarizes the toxic effect of sugar in his book, *Sugar Blues*, when he kicked the habit. Dufty threw all the sugar in his kitchen out and just ate grains and vegetables. He wrote,

> In about forty-eight hours, I was in total agony, overcome with nausea, with a crashing migraine. If pain was a message, this was a long one, very involved, intense but in code. It took hours to break the code. I knew enough about junkies to recognize reluctantly my kinship with them. I was kicking cold turkey, the thing they talked about with such terror. After all, heroin is nothing but a chemical. They take the juice of the poppy and they refine it into opium and then they refine it to morphine and finally to heroin. Sugar is nothing but a chemical. They take the juice of the cane or the beet and

they refine it to molasses and then they refine it to brown sugar and finally to strange white crystals. It's no wonder dope pushers dilute pure heroin with milk sugar—lactose—in order to make their glassine packages a treat to the eye. I was kicking all kinds of chemicals cold turkey—sugar, aspirin, cocaine, caffeine, chlorine, fluorine, sodium, monosodium glutamate, and all those other multisyllabic horrors listed in fine print on the tins and boxes I had just thrown in the trash. I had it very rough for about twenty-four hours, but the morning after was a revelation. I went to sleep with exhaustion, sweating and tremors. I woke up feeling reborn."[1]

You may or may not experience such withdrawals depending on how much you are addicted to sugar. Dufty ate a high carbohydrate diet when he went off sugar, which was at the very least, better than eating a diet full of sugar. Eating a high carbohydrate diet helps reduce the addictive withdrawal symptoms of getting off sugar. Carbohydrate is units of different type sugar. If you eat the 'typical American diet' that includes 149 pounds of sugar a year, addiction to sugar is no doubt the reason many cannot stop eating sugar.

William Dufty wrote on page 175 of his book,

"It is mind boggling today to read through medical histories and other tomes and find again and again that the basic cause of diabetes mellitus is still unknown, that it is chronic and incurable, or that it is due to the failure of the pancreas to secrete an adequate amount of insulin. It's still Greek to the best of them."[2]

In 2003 on the American Diabetes Association's website, when you click on Basic Diabetes Information, you may read this statement:

---

1.   *Sugar Blues*, William Dufty, 1975, Warner Books, Inc, p. 22–3
2.   *ibid.*, p. 77–8

"The cause of diabetes continues to be a mystery, although both genetics and environmental factors such as obesity and lack of exercise appear to play roles."

This gives you an idea of how the mainstream health authorities appear to be clueless to diet's connection with disease. But you do see the connection don't you? The above quote says obesity plays a factor in diabetes.

Medical authorities agree that persons with diabetes are at a higher risk for heart disease. Yet connecting sugar consumption over the years to either disease is overlooked, minimized or lacking by these medical authorities. If you look at a graph published in the book *Sugar Busters!*, it shows how the consumption of sugar has climbed dramatically only in the last couple of centuries. Now compare this with a graph on the dramatic climb of diabetes during this same period, it doesn't take a clinical study to see the connection. The damage of high sugar consumption to a person's body not only effects diseases like diabetes and heart disease but possibly is one of the major factors in many other diseases. Remember 170 million people on this planet have diabetes and the number continues to rise along with increases in world sugar production.

While the USDA's Food Pyramid 'balanced food group' diet limits sugar, the pyramid still blesses sugar consumption in small amounts at the top of the pyramid.

Obesity is now the culprit used by medical authorities as being the factor for several major diseases. Does diet play a factor in obesity? Sugar causes obesity. Reducing sugar in your diet will reduce obesity. Eliminating sugar from your diet promotes health and well being. Eliminating sugar in a rosacean diet controls rosacea.

Weight loss will result when you reduce sugar in your diet. How does this happen? Your body breaks down all food into glucose so that the cells can use the energy and live. Any excess glucose is converted to glycogen ("animal starch") and stored in your liver, muscles and blood to be used if needed. This is a wonderful storehouse of packed energy that can easily be converted back to glucose when needed. There is one problem. The body can only store about 14 ounces of glycogen or about 400 grams.[3] A gram of glucose has four calories. The entire amount of stored glycogen is approximately 1600 to 1800 calories. Since there is limited glycogen storage, if your diet includes a generous amount of sugars and carbohydrate and your glycogen storehouse is full, the excess sugars and carbohydrate will be converted to **FAT** and the body gains weight. The *Rosacea Diet* stops this excess conversion of sugars and carbohydrate into fat, thus resulting in weight loss over time. This is just one of the reasons why sugar should be avoided in your diet not to mention you will feel healthier!

Refined sugar [sucrose] in crystallized form is artificial usually made from either sugar beets or sugarcane. Some may claim that sugar is natural, but would you call the crystallized powder heroin derived from morphine 'natural,' because it is made from the opium of a poppy? Refined table sugar doesn't occur naturally, it is an artificially manufactured process. I toured a sugar plantation and factory in Kauai, Hawaii this year and saw the process how sugar cane is made into raw sugar. Lime is used. What is done to raw sugar to make this product into a pure white crystal? There is no way you can call this natural. It is a manufactured processed artificial sugar reducing the sugar cane plant into an addictive pure white crystal not unlike how the poppy flower is used to make opium into morphine and heroine. This process is a manufacturing artificial process not found in nature. You simply do not find these white crystals called sugar or heroine in nature.

---

3.   *Nutrition For Dummies* ®, 1997, Carol Ann Rinzler, IDG Books Worldwide, Inc., p. 81

You may ask, 'if sugar is so bad for your health, why do the health or *diet authorities* minimize the toxic effects of sugar?' The *Sugar Buster!* authors put it this way on page 36–37 of their book,

> "...Pro-sugar lobbying by sugar growers, cola manufactures and the packaged-food industry has been very effective in influencing our government. What politician wants to tell his constituents they should no longer eat sugar?"

Why do health 'authorities' continue to bless sugar? Another reason may be the quote below:

> "The American Dietetic Association, which trains registered dieticians to direct preparation of hospital and institutional food, has been soundly criticized for its association with the Sugar Association and companies like Coca Cola and M&M Mars. Such groups supply about 15% of the ADA's annual budget..."[4]

Sugar is big business. It permeates the food industry. If you think the tobacco industry is powerful, the sugar industry is just as entrenched powerfully in the world's economy if not more so. Even if it reached the point of a warning label of sugar's toxic effects like the tobacco industry has been forced to use on its product, people will continue to eat sugar just as those who smoke ignore the warning label. Only people who care about their health will be motivated enough to remove sugar from their diet.

There is so much information on the web or in your public library showing the harmful effects of sugar. Just go to any major search engine and type in 'sugar' in the search box and you will be amazed at

---

4. *Nourishing Traditions*, Sally Fallon with Mary G. Enig, Ph.D, New Trends Publishing, 1999, P. 571

the results. Or spend a few hours at your local library. I have chosen some books and these two urls as examples:

Dangers of Sugar
78 Ways Sugar Can Ruin Your Health
http://www.mercola.com/article/sugar/

Refined sugar—the sweetest poison of all
http://www.askwaltstollmd.com/archives/sugar/5283.html
http://www.bcn.net/~stoll/sugarimm.html

There are a number of articles and books you may read on this subject which are listed below or can be found on the web:

Pure, White and Deadly, John Yudkin, Viking, 186, Penguin, 188, Davis-Poynter Ltd; ASIN: 070670006

Sweet and Dangerous: The New Facts About the Sugar You Eat As a Cause of Heart Disease, Diabetes, and Other Killers. by John Yudkin

Metabolic Effects of Utilizable Dietary Carbohydrate by Sheldon Reiser (Editor) (Hardcover—August 1982)

The Saccharine Disease: Conditions Caused by the taking of Refined Carbohydrate, such as sugar and white flour by T. L. Cleave

Dismantling a Myth: The Role of Fat and Carbohydrate in Our Diet by Wolfgang Lutz

Refined Carbohydrate Foods and Disease: Some Implications of Dietary Fiber by D. Burkitt

Are you beginning to understand that *sugar suffice is not nice*!

Sugars to Avoid

This chapter should be used to refer when you are using the thirty-day diet plan for vegetarians or omnivores. The Nutrition Facts Label appearing on all USA products sold in America can be used to find the total amount of carbohydrate in a product. If you are in another country hopefully there is something on the product that lists something. There is also a list of ingredients usually on every USA product that may list sugars used. Both of these can be used to figure out if sugar is in a product, first the **Nutrition Facts Label** and second, the LIST OF INGREDIENTS. Keep in mind the food process industry has figured out ways to hide the sugar in a product. You have to be smart to figure whether a product has sugar in it to avoid the product for thirty days. Of course, you as the *diet authority* can eat as much sugar as you want, but I am suggesting you avoid this entire list of sugars for thirty days to see if you control your rosacea and feel healthier. At the end of the thirty days you may decide to avoid sugar for life!

I think I have compiled one of the longest lists of sugars used by the processed food industry that keeps finding new ways to add sugar to your life. This list is by no means complete because as soon as I publish this current list I find new ones. What I suggest is that you at least read the list. This will give you an idea of how invasive sugar has become in the processed food industry in all its various forms. After all, carbohydrate is simply different units of sugar so it is only a matter of breaking some food down into a simple sugar to be added to a product so it tastes sweeter and you buy it. If you find one not on this list, please join the Rosacea Diet Users Support Group and post it so I can add it to a future revision of this book. I also keep a current list of the Sugars to Avoid in a file on the yahoo group site for you to read.

SUGAR TO AVOID

(For thirty days avoid the following sugars which may appear on any list of ingredients)

Agave Nectar
Arabinose
Apricot nectar
Barley malt
Beet Sugar
Blackstrap Molasses
Brown Sugar
Cane Juice
Cane Sugar
Corn Sweetner
Corn Syrup
Corn solids
Dark brown sugar molasses
Date Sugar
Dextrose (an optical isomer of glucose which is dextrorotatory)
Evaporated cane juice
Fruit Juice Concentrate (any type fruit—apple, pear, grape, etc.)
Fructooligosaccharides
Fructose (CH2OH(CHOH)3COCH2OH)
Galactose; (C6H12O6)
Glucose (C6H12O6)
Glycogen
High Fructose Corn Syrup (HFCS)
Honey
Invert Sugar (50:50 fructose-glucose)

Lactose (C12H22O11)
Levulose
Maltose
Maltodextrin
Mannose
Maple Syrup
Molasses
Monosaccharides
Muscovado (Natural light brown muscovado sugar)
Organic sugar
Organic powdered sugar
Papaya Nectar
Peach Nectar
Polycose
Polydextrose
Polysaccarides
Powdered sugar
Raffinose
Rapadura
Raw Sugar
Rice syrup
Sorghum
Starch
Stachyose
Sucanat
Sucrose (C12H22O11)
Sugar Cane Juice
Sugar Cane natural organic Sucanat
Sugar crystals
Syrup (any type no matter what)
Turbinado Sugar
Turbino

Unsulfured Molasses
Xylose

All Sugar Substitutes are to be avoided for thirty days such as:

Acesulfame-K
Acesulfame Potassium
Alitame
Aspartame
Cyclamates
Equal
Lo Han
Luo Han Guo Fruit extract
Neotame
Nutrisweet
Saccharin
Splenda
Stevia
Stevia plus fiber
Sucralose
Sweet and Slender

Sugar Alcohols to avoid:

Hydrogenated Starch Hydrolysates (HSH)
Isomalt
Lactitol
Maltitol
Mannitol
Sorbitol
Xylitol

For more information on sugar substitutes go to this url >

http://www.cfsan.fda.gov/~dms/fdsugar.html

http://www.aspartemekills.com

The sugar alcohols-xylitol, mannitol, and sorbitol have some calories or carbohydrate that slightly increase blood glucose level. Avoid anything that says 'syrup' whether corn syrup or 'any' syrup! Some sugar substitutes may have carbohydrate so look at the Nutrition Facts Label and note any carbohydrate or sugar grams. Watch out for maltitol and corn syrup solids. **NO SUGAR SUBSTITUES** even if it has ZERO sugars or carbohydrate for thirty days, **NONE**. It doesn't matter whatever name it is called, whether calorie-free sweeteners like Nutrisweet, Splenda, Equal, aspartame, saccharin, and acesulfame-K**, NO SUGAR SUBSTITUTES**—AFTER the thirty days you can experiment with sugar substitutes all you want. You will figure out if your health suffers by this simple thirty-day experiment of avoiding sugar substitutes. You will know if you can use them or not when you try them again, no matter what the health authorities say about the safety of these sugar substitutes. Remember that you are the *diet authority*, not anyone else.

Some have found that certain sugar substitutes trigger allergic reactions or cause health problems. The real reason for no sugar substitutes for thirty days is so you can taste sugar in your food and drink, to be able to detect it! If you are sprinkling or adding sugar substitutes to your food or drink during the 30 Day Diet Plan, there is no way for you to be able to taste if sugar is somehow present in any of the food or drink you consume. Consequently you will then be more sensitive to the taste of sugar in your food or drink to avoid it for the 30 Days.

AFTER the thirty days, you may experiment all you want. First, prove to yourself that the *Rosacea Diet* does CONTROL your rosacea and helps you feel healthier! You will be surprised at how sensitive you become in detecting sugar in your food and drink and how it creeps into processed food and drink. Most sugar substitutes are processed from sugar and are just as unhealthy for you as sugar, if not more so. What do you think the long-term health risks are from sugar substitutes? You will find out if you use them.

So if you have to use a sugar substitute **AFTER the 30-day Rosacea Diet plan**, I recommend **Stevia**, a natural leaf that is 300 times sweeter than sugar with zero carbohydrate grams found in health stores. Who knows what the long-term use of **Stevia** may do to you but you may be able to use it instead of sugar or sugar substitutes and be healthier? So Stevia is my recommendation and you will just have to live with the health consequences. Some have claimed that Stevia poses no health risks. One thing I have found with Stevia is less is more. The more Stevia the worse it tastes. The less Stevia the better it tastes. You can find out more information on Stevia by typing in Stevia into any search engine and boom you get more information that you can handle.

Sweet Leaf Stevia Plus Fiber contains a packet that has less than 1 gram of carbohydrate per serving. More info at >

http://www.steviaplus.com

An alternative is Sweet and Slender Natural sweetener made from fructose and Luo Han Guo fruit extract that contains less than one gram of carbohydrate per packet. Both of these products can be found at the following urls >
http://www.sweetandslender.com
http://www.wisdomherbs.com

Another product made by Renew Life is SweetLife made from fructose, Lo Han and fructooligosaccharides which has one gram of carbohydrate per gram serving.

My recommendation is avoid all other sugar substitutes and sugar for the rest of your life but since you are the *diet authority*, you choose. It may be possible that some of the sugar substitutes mentioned above might not pose any health problems but I don't recommend eating 149 pounds of the product in a year. Moderation in sugar substitutes is obvious.

Vitamins and Supplements

Daily Vitamin Supplements Suggested

Acidophilus (40,000,000 CFU three times a day or more)
Vitamin A—25,000 IU
High Potency B Complex—1 tab/capsule
Flush Free Niacin [B-3] (Inositol Hexanicotinate)—100 mg
Pantothenic Acid [B-5]—100mg
B-6—50 mg
B-12—250 mcg.
Beta Carotene—25,000 IU
Calcium—at least 1000 mg
Zinc—15 mg
Vitamin C [at least 500—suggest 1000 to 3000 mg] (*Ester-C*™ recommended)
Vitamin D—400 I.U.
Vitamin E—400 I.U.
Evening Primrose—1000 mg.
Fish Oil—1000 mg
Grape Seed Extract—50 mg
Glucosamine Complex—1.5 g
L-Lysine—1000 mg
Magnesium—399 mg
MSM (Methylsulfonylmethane)—1000 mg
Multivitamin—1 tab
Pantothenic Acid—500 mg
Potassium—1100 mg
Selenium—200 mcg

These are the minimum suggested

More vitamins are your choice. By taking vitamins, it will help curb your appetite for sweets. And in a few weeks you will notice the difference they can make in your life. My personal theory is that we need the extra vitamin supplements since the processed food in our diet lacks nutrients and we need the boost since an insulin dominant metabolism has been leaching our vitamins and minerals. If you decide to take these suggestions always consume vitamins and supplements at breakfast with your food. If you take some vitamins at night, you may not sleep well, so try to take them at breakfast or lunch, always with food. There is some controversy with vitamins, and I don't want to debate on this subject. If you have an issue with any of the above suggestions, remember that the above vitamins/minerals are just a suggestion. I buy most of my vitamins at Wal-Mart or Costco. Some complain that vitamins are costly but give no thought to the cost of junk food, candy or milk shakes. If you cut out the sugar and junk food for thirty days the money you save should more than compensate the investment of vitamin and mineral supplements I suggest. You will not believe how the vitamins and minerals suggested would improve your health and give you the boost you need for energy unless you try it. Whatever the cost, it is only for thirty days and after that you can decide yourself if the money you spent on vitamins and minerals was worth it. To give you an idea of the cost of this my wife and I spend about $75 a month for two people on vitamins and supplements in 2003. How much do you spend for dinner out at a nice restaurant? So you can't sacrifice one restaurant meal during this month you are trying the *Rosacea Diet*? If money is still the issue then do the best you can with vitamins. The amount of vitamins I suggest taking doesn't have to be set in stone. You can alter the suggestions according to what brand you buy and figure it out for your situation.

I also suggest you take the following vitamins just before bed with a glass of water:

Acidophilus (40,000,000 CFU)

L-Lysine—500 mg

Calcium—1000 mg

Magnesium—399 mg

Zinc—15 mg

Potassium—1100 mg

Vitamin C—1000 mg. (*Ester-C*™ recommended)

Water

Water is essential for human survival. We get water from the food and drink we consume. What is the minimum amount of water essential for good health? There is considerable variation here due to individual sweating rates, body size and weight, heat and humidity, and running speed, and other factors.[1] However it is generally believed that for the average adult two liters of water a day is recommended.[2] Your individual condition determines how much water you may need to lose weight and feel healthier. But you may not be getting enough water with your current diet and I recommend more water than you may be currently drinking.

During the thirty-days of the *Rosacea Diet* I suggest drinking at least eight glasses of twelve-ounces of water and if possible drinking ten glasses. Most health authorities recommend drinking eight glasses of eight ounces of water per day. I prefer twelve ounces because you can visualize a twelve-ounce container. An eight-ounce container is not easily visualized since they are rare. I think you need more water for health or to lose weight.

---

1. "The primary determinant of maintenance water requirement appears to be metabolic (Holliday and Segar, 1957), but the actual estimation of water requirement is highly variable and quite complex. Because the water requirement is the amount necessary to balance the insensible losses (which can vary markedly) and maintain a tolerable solute load for the kidneys (which may vary with dietary composition and other factors), it is impossible to set a general water requirement." Source >
http://books.nap.edu/books/0309046335/html/249.html#pagetop

2. http://www.i-medreview.com/articles_html/
nutritionwellness/essnutrients.html

Some may be concerned about drinking this much water, which is a valid concern. You can not be drinking too much water unless you have a disease state like kidney, heart disease, or some other condition. I have explained in my legal disclaimer that you should not begin this diet without consulting your physician. Excess water normally will be passed out of the body by urinating, sweating, defecating, and exhaling thereby preventing fluid retention. A condition known as hyponatremia[3]—sometimes called water intoxication—is caused when levels of sodium in the blood drop to dangerously low levels. However, this condition is rare and usually found in extreme cases, such as long distance runners who drink copious amounts of water without replenishing sodium or electrolytes resulting in the body's salt and water levels getting dangerously out of balance. It leads to swelling of the brain and leakage of fluid into the lungs. Remember that this condition is rare and extreme.

The range I suggest is between 96 ounces of water per day to a maximum of 120 ounces. This amounts to between two and a half liters to a little over three liters of water per day. For thirty days this usually will pose no health problems. If you have some health condition causing you water retention or some other health concern discuss your water intake and diet with your health care practitioner. Our kidneys are equipped to efficiently process fifteen liters of water a day. That's equivalent to drinking about sixty glasses of water! I am not recommending sixty glasses of water. Excess water we take in that is not needed is usually passed out as urine within a few hours if everything is working satisfactorily.

---

3.   "Toxicity results from the ingestion of water at a rate beyond the capacity of the kidneys to excrete the extra load, resulting in hyposmolarity. Such a condition is rarely observed in a normal healthy adult. The manifestations usually include a gradual mental dulling, confusion, coma, convulsion, and even death." Source > http://books.nap.edu/books/0309046335/html/250.html#pagetop

By most current dietetic standards, the guideline is that most healthy adults normally require approximately three quarts of fluid each day. Half of the liquid comes from food and the other half from what you drink. Drinking 8 to 12 glasses a day of eight-ounce containers should be sufficient for keeping your system in good working order. But I recommend more since I think you need to flush your system to control your rosacea and feel healthier when changing over from an insulin dominant metabolism to a glucagon dominant one.

In the thirty-day plan I have suggested when to drink a glass of 12 ounces of water in ten suggested times a day for each day of the diet. Not juice, soft drinks, just water! If you can't drink that much water, remember this is just a suggestion and you are the *diet authority* and can drink whatever amount you want or drink the amount recommended by your health practitioner. You may find that drinking the amount of water I suggest will help you lose weight, feel healthier, and control your rosacea.

Puzzling Pyramids

Before the USDA came out with its famous Food Guide Pyramid in 1992, the typical American ate 40% Fat, 15% Protein, and 45% Carbohydrate.[1] If you like, go to this url and check out the Food Guide and try to figure out the percentages that the government recommended to the public in 1992 >

http://www.pueblo.gsa.gov/cic_text/food/food-pyramid/main.htm

If you can figure it out you are one smart cookie. The only percentage mentioned is the famous 30% fat figure. That is why I call it a puzzling pyramid. Who can understand it? Servings? What does that mean? My wife may serve her plate and I would still be hungry if I ate her servings. What percentage of protein should I eat? What percentage of carbohydrate should I eat? Another puzzle is how the USDA Pyramid breaks food up. It breaks all food into six categories:

Fats, Oils and Sweets—Use Sparingly
Milk, Yogurt, Cheese Group—2 to 3 Servings
Meat, Poultry, Fish, Dry beans, Eggs & Nuts Group—2 to 3 Servings
Vegetable Group—3 to 5 Servings
Fruit Group—2 to 4 Servings
Grain Group—5–11 Servings

Ok, where is a McDonald's hamburger in this pyramid? What about a pepperoni pizza? Are you puzzled? The brochure that the government

---

1. *Scientific American*, January 2003, *Rebuilding the Food Pyramid*, Walter C. Willett and Meir J. Stampfer

provides to explain this pyramid is more puzzling. If you note at the top of the pyramid that fat is to be used sparingly yet the brochure says that your total fat can be up to 30%. Is that confusing to you? That makes this pyramid contradictory if the tiny top of the pyramid allows 30% of your total caloric intake. I can make it more puzzling but you can at least see why most Americans ignore this Pyramid. The bottom line is that the USDA Food Guide Pyramid is approximately 60% Carbohydrate, 25% Fat, and 15% Protein.

As Newsweek magazine pointed out, Americans ignore this pyramid and eat what they want and have chosen to eat more sweets and meat. The typical American Diet works out to approximately 75% Carbohydrate, 15% Protein, and 10% Fat. What the USDA Food Guide Pyramid accomplished was to change the American way of eating before 1992 from eating 40% fat to 10% and instead of eating more protein everyone ate more carbohydrate.

The USDA is planning on revising the Food Guide Pyramid and it is reported to be released sometime in 2004.[2] There are other pyramids like the NEW FOOD GUIDE PYRAMID mentioned in the preceding *Newsweek* magazine article, the Mediterranean Food Pyramid, the Asian Food Pyramid and probably others you may have heard of. I still find them all puzzling. What I find easier to understand is not pyramids but percentages. You can imagine the three food groups in your mind right now, can't you? So let's discuss percentages.

Just about all the health authorities say you can eat up to 30% Fat. So starting with this as a base lets figure out in our minds what should be the percentages of proteins and fats. An easy way to do this is simply divide the three groups into thirds and each group would be 33 per cent. Based on the current nutritional research splitting it three ways

2.   *Scientific American*, January 2003, *Rebuilding the Food Pyramid*, Walter C. Willett and Meir J. Stampfer

equally is better than the typical American diet which has raised obesity.

The authorities point out that the MINIMUM requirement of protein to survive is somewhere between 50 to 100 grams. You think you just want to eat the minimum, or should we eat more for better health? Duh? We need protein. You need protein to heal, build, and grow. We don't *need* carbohydrate. Carbohydrate is like dessert that makes life enjoyable. We need to *maximize* our protein intake, not maximize our carbohydrate. A good goal is to eat at least 50% protein, 20% for carbohydrate. Doesn't that make sense? If you raise the protein even higher it won't hurt, in fact you will heal! Rosaceans need protein to heal their rosacea.

The thirty-day *Rosacea Diet* in this book (based on a 2000 calorie a day diet) is:

64% PROTEIN—30% FAT—6% CARBOHYDRATE

The Rosacea Diet is *extreme* for thirty days to change your insulin dominant metabolism over to a glucagon dominant one to control your rosacea. AFTER the thirty days you can then experiment all you want with the percentages of the three basic food groups. The thirty-day *Rosacea diet* is to prove you can control your rosacea and feel healthier with a high protein diet.

The debate over these percentages will go on and on. You are the *diet authority* and you can decide your own percentages AFTER the thirty-day diet plan. Most *Rosacea Diet* users still eat a high protein diet and many discuss how they are doing this in the *Rosacea Diet* Users Support Group. The other debate is what protein, fat and carbohydrate to eat. Fix in mind that protein should be at the top of the percentage, not carbohydrate. That is what should be in your mind and the puzzling pyramids can stay in Egypt where they ought to be.

Alcohol

Are you aware that some beer and wine contain added sugar? Most alcohol contains high concentrations of sugar. Alcohol manufactures are not required to list the ingredients so you will never see it on a label. Alcohol is made mostly with sugar. Lots of it. Distilled spirits are made from lots of sugar and good wine has high amounts of fructose. Beer is loaded with maltose or adulterated with sucrose. <u>So for one month no alcohol</u>, period. After the thirty days, you can return to your favorite alcohol. Also, if you are an alcoholic you may find out during this 30-day period you have a problem with it by avoiding it.

Wine and Beer are the highest in sugar content, while the distilled spirits have fewer calories. AFTER the 30 day Diet Plan you may discover how much alcohol you can consume without weight gain and feel healthy. The sugar in alcohol is what you need to avoid for 30 days to control your rosacea and feel healthier. To give you an idea about the carbohydrate gram count in alcohol, 12 fl. oz. of regular beer contains 13.7 grams of carbohydrate, 12 fl. oz of table wine contains 14.7 grams of carbohydrate, while distilled spirits (hard liquors such as whisky, Scotch, vodka, bourbon, gin, etc,) ANY PROOF of 1 fl. oz contain only a trace of carbohydrate! So if you consume alcohol AFTER THE THIRTY DAYS beer and wine may increase your weight. The distilled spirits you may find may not increase weight. Moderation is the key for good health.

I recently discovered Michelob Ultra that only has 2.6 grams of carbohydrate per 12 fluid ounces. But you have to wait until your thirty days are up. I imagine if this beer becomes popular there will be many other beers touting low carbohydrate and we can be thankful for that. But you may find that you may have to stay away from beer and wine altogether and stick to the distilled spirits with no sugar added to the drink.

What you do with alcohol after the thirty days is your choice. It may be that alcohol is related to some health problems you are having and by not consuming alcohol for thirty days you may discover some relief.

Remember to avoid alcohol for thirty days. You can do it. At the end of the thirty days you can have that drink! Remember that you are the *diet authority*.

Prove it to Yourself

Avoid eating or drinking sugar or sugar substitutes for a month to see for yourself. It will probably be the most difficult month you have ever experienced. This is not an over-statement. Just try it. Not eating sugar in your diet for just three days will show you how difficult it is. Two weeks without sugar is like an alcoholic trying to quit drinking for the same period. What is really amusing, is that most reputable authorities think that sugar is not an addiction. But just try not eating sugar for two weeks and tell me that you are not addicted to sugar! I have been off sugar for years and I still CRAVE it. So don't think this will be easy.

The typical American diet includes a generous percentage of refined sugar. Sugar occurs naturally in many foods, such as fruit, which contains fructose. Trying to find food that you like, containing no sugar, is very difficult at first since you may not have given it much thought and especially if you eat a lot of processed food or eat in restaurants/fast food chains. Most processed food has sugar, as you will discover. However, you can still live a meaningful life without sugar. It can be done, many have done it, and you can too. I will tell you more on how you can get help avoiding sugar, and how to join the *Rosacea Diet* Users Support Group for encouragement. But for now, just try to avoid eating sugar and carbohydrate for a month and eating a diet high in protein to see if your health gets better and if you lose weight.

During this one-month test, drink plenty of WATER. Please read the chapter on *Water*.

Also, be sure to get enough VITAMINS in your diet, which will curb your appetite for sweets. Supplemental vitamins help so read the chapter on *Vitamins and Supplements.*

Get plenty of rest. If you are under a lot of stress, this will not help your diet, so don't add to your stress by overdoing it. Try to pick a thirty-day period that is stress free. Don't start this diet if you are under stress. The ideal thirty-day period to begin this diet is a long vacation. But even if you do not have the luxury to avoid stress, you will find that to the extent you avoid sugar in your diet, you should notice some commensurate improvement in your rosacea.

Exercise is necessary. You know all the authorities say exercise is needed for health. As *Newsweek*[1] puts it,

> "Diet alone, however, isn't enough. You also need to get moving. That doesn't mean you have to become an exercise maniac. A half-hour of brisk walking a day can dramatically lower your risk of chronic disease. The payoff for all this effort is huge: a longer, healthier life."

You know this is true. I know that exercise can be a rosacea trigger. But get real, I am not advocating a strenuous work out during the thirty days. Some moderate exercise. At the very least go on regular walks. Finding the time, motivation and will power to do this and to change your diet is the issue. You are not only the *diet authority* but also the authority of your body that needs to get moving.

---

1.   *Newsweek*, January 20, 2003, p.45

Why Do I Still Have Rosacea?

The answer is that this diet does not cure rosacea, it only controls it. If you take prescription medication to control rosacea you still have rosacea. What I have learned from those who say the *Rosacea Diet* has not helped them is because they did not reduce their carbohydrate intake to less than 30 grams a day. This is not always the case, but it is the number one reason. They simply cannot stick to a high protein diet. Why? The will power necessary to avoid sugar and carbohydrate for thirty days is tremendous. Another reason is they cheated occasionally or didn't reduce their sugar intake enough due to carelessness. Some sprinkle sugar substitutes into their food and drink thinking this is ok, but cannot tell that sugar has crept into their food or drink and did not detect it since their taste buds are not sugar sensitive and ate more than 30 grams of carbohydrate a day unknowingly. That is why I recommend no sugar substitutes for thirty days so you can detect sugar in your food and drink. <u>AFTER</u> the thirty days you can experiment with sugar substitutes, just like any thing else you want.

You might not be aware of how sugar gets into your diet. And remember this isn't a controlled study, it is simply your ability to avoid sugar, in all its forms, artificial refined sugar [sucrose] or natural sugar, whether it is sucrose, fructose, lactose, maltose, glucose, etc. Do you actually read the ingredients written on the package, bottle, can, or wrap that your food or drink contains? Even "sugarless" products sometimes contain other sources of sugar like brown sugar, fructose, corn syrup, honey, molasses, maltose, glucose, or some synonym for sugar. The food labels have all sorts of ways to hide sugar. The processed food manufacturers have found so many ways to keep some form of sugar in a product that you have to become a detective to find it. Absolutely no honey or maple syrup! And in order for you to be able to detect anything sweet in your food for thirty days, <u>please don't eat any sugar substitute</u> since you will not detect if sugar is still present in the food or drink you are consuming. I know this is hard, but your taste buds need to be sensitive to anything sweet and artificial sweeteners mask any sugar that may be present. <u>Avoiding sugar substitutes solves this problem for thirty days!</u> Does this take motivation and will power? Not many have either one, so you have to ask yourself if you as the *diet authority* can simply do this for thirty days? There is light at the end of this tunnel! A clear face. It is worth the effort. It is only thirty days.

Reading the Nutrition Facts Label

Nutrition Facts Label on any packaging lists **TOTAL CARBOHY-DRATE**, and then lists under this "**Sugars**" and/or "**Sugar Alcohols**" and the total grams per serving. This is the where you find sugar in the ingredients, even if it is hidden in the list by some other name not mentioned in the list above. I keep finding new ones. So if you find any that I have not listed in the chapter, **Sugars to Avoid**, let me know so I can add it to the list. More information on this can be found at this url >

http://www.stanford.edu/group/ketodiet/cholabel.html

Also, watch out for "SUGAR FREE" or 'NO SUGAR ADDED!' This only means no sucrose or NO MORE SUGAR added since it usually CONTAINS some form of sugar hidden in the ingredients in a different form! An interesting link you may check is "The Sugar Free Hoax" > http://www.wilstar.net/sugarfree

The way the **Nutrition Facts Label** lists food is the order of amounts. The most listed first and the least listed last. So if the sugar word shows up near the first of the list the product is loaded with sugar! If the sugar word shows up in the list at all, avoid the product for thirty days. Learning to read this label will really improve your health and you will lose weight. The USDA has some helpful links if you still have questions about this label.

http://www.cfsan.fda.gov/label.html
http://www.nal.usda.gov/fnic/cgi-bin/nut_search.pl

If an item contains less than 1 gram of sugar or carbohydrate in a serv-ing, for example, dextrose, the Nutrition Food Label will say Zero Car-bohydrate. The dextrose is less than one gram per serving or unit. The Nutrition Facts Label is where you find the carbohydrate and sugar content in any food or drink. This is the best way to discover the car-bohydrate or sugar content. The ingredient list can be misleading and the processed food industry is good at hiding sugar on ingredient lists and packaging statements. The one good thing the government health authorities did was requiring the Nutrition Facts Label to know the truth about a product. The list of ingredients can be helpful but the real information is found in the **Nutrition Facts Label**. An excellent book to count carbohydrate grams is, *Dr. Atkins' New Carbohydrate Gram Counter*, 1996, M. Evans and Company, Inc, New York, New York. You can obtain this book at this url along with other diet books >
http://www.rosacea-diet/html/dietbooks.html

How Can I Get Help?

Join the **Rosacea Diet Users Support Group** at yahoo groups by sending an email to this address:

rosacea-diet-users-support-group-subscribe@yahoogroups.com

If you join *Rosacea Diet* Users Support Group there is a database of **recipes** available. There are links to related web sites to check but another chapter explains about this group with detailed information.

Also there are five books which I recommend as additional reading which will actually help you and may change your eating habits for life! Here is the list:

Sugar Blues by William Dufty, 1975, Warner Books, Inc
Sugar Busters! By H. Leighton Steward, Dr. Morrison C. Bethea, Dr. Samuel S. Andrews, and Dr. Luis A Balart, 15, *Sugar Busters!*, LLC, 1995
Protein Power by Michael R. Eades, M.D. and Mary Dan Eades, M.D., 16, Bantam Books, 1996
Dr. Atkins' New Carbohydrate Gram Counter by Robert C. Atkins, 1996, M.D., M. Evans and Company, Inc
Dr. Atkin's New Diet Revolution by Robert C. Atkins, M.D., 2001, Avon

These books will verify the need to find a diet avoiding sugar in all its forms. Like I said, this isn't going to be easy, especially if you eat out a lot. You may need additional support. You already know that all the food you eat is eventually converted to glucose so your cells can use the energy from what you eat. Your body takes a lot more time and energy to convert protein to glucose through protein synthesis, which is discussed in another chapter. By reading these books you will also discover a lot of information which will help you understand the role insulin and glucagon has on your body. Glucagon is a hormone secreted by the pancreas that helps regulate blood sugar and metabolize stored fat. Could it be possible that eating sugar over the years taxes the pancreas upsetting the hormonal balance in our immune system and we need to stimulate glucagon in our bodies to get healthy? Insulin dominance in our body as a result of eating too much sugar in the diet over the years should be replaced with a glucagon dominance in our body by avoiding sugar and eating a high protein diet. Could it be that sugar is just a poison that over many years of consumption causes vascular disorders or cancers? Mr. Dufty, in *Sugar Blues* did not discuss the role glucagon has on the body when he wrote his book in 1975, and didn't understand that a diet high in protein is preferable, but instead encouraged a diet high in carbohydrate, which has been popular for years. Dufty's diet, or a high carbohydrate diet will increase blood glucose levels, so I recommend the diet mentioned in *Protein Power* as my preference, but the diet in *Sugar Busters!* is useful. However, Mr. Dufty's book on sugar is the premier source of information on the history of sugar, its sordid past and its unhealthy effects, including the sugar blues. All these books are currently available and can easily be obtained by going online to this site:

http://rosacea-diet.com/html/dietbooks.html

You will also find on this web page some other suggested diet books that will help you find recipes avoiding sugar and carbohydrate to help you. As I said, there are thousands of diet books out there, but I have selected some that are in harmony with the *Rosacea Diet* and you might find some interesting reading.

And there is one more book I suggest you purchase for a complete knowledge of rosacea treatment:

Beating Rosacea—Vascular, Ocular & Acne Forms, A Must-have Guide to Understanding & Treating Rosacea, Dr. Geoffrey Nase, Ph.D. Microvascular Physiologist, 2001, Nase Publications, www.drnase.com

At my web there are listed all the publications known that are available to rosaceans at this url >
http://www.rosacea-diet.com/html/books.html

If there are any new ones they will be posted at the above site.

Ten Suggestions for the Thirty Day Diet Plan

1. Do not eat sugar, sucrose, maltose, lactose, glucose, fructose, or sugar substitutes such as saccharin, cyclamates, aspartame, ace-sulfame-K or any natural sugar substitute, just for thirty days—See the chapter **Sugars to Avoid.**

2. Do not eat carbohydrate or starches unless specifically mentioned in the 30-Day *Diet* Plan—Limit your total carbohydrate intake to 30 grams or less! Read the Nutrition Facts Label on all foods and drinks to determine carbohydrate gram content and **DO NOT EXCEED 30 GRAMS PER DAY!**

    An excellent source for counting carbohydrate grams is found in the chapter on **Reading the Nutrition Label.**

3. Do not smoke or use tobacco[1] for thirty days

4. Drink EIGHT 12 oz. glasses of water every day (TEN glasses are recommended)

5. Take plenty of vitamins—see chapter on **Vitamin & Mineral Supplements**

6. Get plenty of rest and sleep

---

1. **"an average of 5 percent sugar is added to cigarettes**, up to 20 per cent in cigars, and as much as 40 per cent in pipe tobacco, mostly in the form of molasses and such…flue-cured tobacco can contain as much as 20 percent sugar by weight….sugar (sucrose) is added to air-cured tobacco during the blending process…"—from *Sugar Blues* by William Dufty, 1975 Warner Books, p. 190, 192

7. Do not consume ANY ALCOHOL for 30 days—see chapter on **Alcohol**

8. Always remember this is a 30-day test to see if you lose weight or feel healthier, remember, this is a test—at the end of the thirty days you can return to eating whatever you want!

9. Do not cheat

10. Eat protein, protein, **PROTEIN, as much as you want**, and don't worry about any of the fat that comes with the protein—You won't go hungry on this diet since you can eat all the protein you want!

30 Days—30 Grams of Carbohydrate a Day—No Sugar

The *Rosacea Diet* 30-Day Diet Plan is for only thirty days. After you have proven to yourself that this diet works, you can then eat whatever you want, or modify this diet any way you think best. The *Rosacea Diet* is simply the beginning of a new life style diet that works for you. Go ahead and eat all those sugar delights you crave and see your rosacea return. If you wish to control your rosacea and feel healthier, you can go back on the *Rosacea Diet* or modify it any way you want with additional carbohydrate till you find the diet you can control your control your weight or feel healthy with your eating habits. Remember the 8th suggestion, "Always remember this is a 30 day test to see if this controls your weight and feel healthier, remember, this is a test." If the test proves true, you can then decide for yourself how you are going to control your weight and feel healthy with your diet any way you want after the test.

You should eat less than 30 grams of carbohydrate a day during the thirty day *Rosacea Diet Plan.* If you eat more than 30 grams of carbohydrate per day, your rosacea may not improve. You need to learn how to count your carbs! Once source is *Sugar Busters!* which is an excellent source for counting carbs and understanding the glycemic index, which is discussed in a later chapter. 30 days, 30 grams of carbohydrate and NO SUGAR of any kind.

By the way when you eat salt, be sure to check the box of salt and see if DEXTROSE is added to your salt. I suggest sea salt or at the very least kosher salt. Sea Salt is better for you than the processed salt with dextrose added. Even if you find processed salt without dextrose or sugar it is still refined so much that all the essential minerals are removed. If you do a search on sea salt or the brand Celtic Salt you will find some interesting information why sea salt is better than the processed salt with or without dextrose. One url to consider is >

http://www.elementsofwellness.com/celticsalt.htm

There are other sites that discuss the advantages of sea salt over processed table salt which has all the minerals removed that your body needs. Did you know that salt is an essential element the body needs and yet the health authorities have made salt just as evil as fat? Why would they make salt, an essential mineral, a bad guy?

30-Day Meat Eaters Diet Plan

The next thirty days will prove whether you can control your weight and feel healthier with your diet if you stick to this diet and don't cheat! The good thing about this diet is that you can eat as much as you want of the protein listed each day! You just have to limit your carbohydrate to 30 grams a day. All you have to do is avoid any sugar, syrups, honey, sugar substitutes, carbohydrate, starches, breads, grains, or fruits not specifically mentioned in the diet. And NO tobacco, because sugar is in your tobacco. Your total carbohydrate intake for EACH day should be 30 grams or less during this thirty day *Rosacea Diet* plan [remember the Second Suggestion].

No matter if you are a vegetarian or a meat eater, avoid raisins, bananas, all fruits, fruit juices, parsnips, honey, carrots, corn/corn-flakes, millet, beets, white rice, pasta, plain crackers, all types of white flour, or any potatoes (any color). All these foods easily convert to glucose and should be avoided for thirty days.

Meat eaters should **AVOID ALL GRAINS** for the thirty-day diet plan. After the thirty days, you can eat as much grain as you want. Grain, of course, includes all bread, pasta, etc., which have too many carbohydrate grams during this thirty-day period. AFTER the thirty days, you can begin experimenting with grains to see your weight return or health problems come back.

Eating just a small amount of catsup, or chocolate, or tablespoon of ice cream is cheating! That nice juicy apple is loaded with fructose, so don't cheat! If your rosacea is severe, it will take a month or more before you notice any improvement. But stick to the Thirty-Day *Diet* Plan and see the results for yourself.

Nuts are acceptable for snacks, peanuts being the first choice, which contain 5 grams carbs), but other nuts may be better for health, so I recommend mixed nuts containing NO PEANUTS. If you have no issues with peanuts, go ahead and eat them but count the carbohydrate gram content and include this in the total for the day. Eat no more than 30 grams of carbohydrate a day including the peanuts! Peanuts may produce an allergy in you if you eat too many so be forewarned. It is possible that you may have a peanut allergy check this web site:

http://www.skincarecampaign.org/peanutall.htm

So you better be careful with peanuts. I have found that mixed nuts containing NO PEANUTS work better for me but during this 30-day period you have to keep your nuts to a minimum. For example, 3 tablespoons of mixed nuts without peanuts (or 28 grams) contain 7 grams of carbohydrate. You can only eat 30 grams of carbohydrate a day. Don't go nuts! If you have to have something sweet, the only fruit allowed to eat is avocados and grapefruits, which aren't sweet, so if you have to, I allow dried apricots, but don't eat more than TWO BITES a day! Two halves of dried apricots contain 5 grams carbs. I have found that sugar substitutes should be avoided during this thirty-day diet plan.

Snacks that you can substitute during the 30-day test are as follows: Nuts, sunflower seeds, pork rinds, lean meat slices, any cheese, almond butter without sugar, celery with cream cheese, dried apricot slices, jerky containing no sugar, hard boiled egg, peanut butter without sugar, WASA Original Crispbread Light Rye (each cracker is 6 grams of carbohydrate/1 Gram Protein). I prefer Ryvita crackers to WASA. Remember to count the total grams per day of carbohydrate of your snacks and meals to 30 grams or less per day as I have mentioned many times.

Your total carbohydrate intake per day should not exceed 30 grams, including snacks. Count those carbs! Eat as much protein as you want and don't worry about any of the fat during this 30-day period. Remember that this is only for 30 days to see if you can lose weight and feel healthy.

During the thirty days you may substitute a protein (i.e. meat, fish, chicken) with another protein. You can modify it to fit your situation. The thirty-day suggestions will give you an idea of how to reduce your carbohydrate to 30 grams a day and eat AS MUCH PROTEIN AS YOU WANT. Yes, I said you could eat as much protein as you want. You just limit the carbohydrate to 30 grams a day. You may substitute a carbohydrate with another carbohydrate as long as you keep within the 30-gram limit per day.

No sugar in sausage which may not be easy to find, but try to find it. If you cannot find sugarless sausage, substitute sugarless bacon, which usually is easier to obtain. By the way, after the 30 days, you may be able to tolerate bacon, sausage or ham whether it is sugar cured or not, you will just have to experiment. But during the thirty days of the diet, do not eat sugar-cured bacon, sausage, ham, or any sugar-cured meat.

You may add heavy cream to the black coffee or tea during the thirty-day diet whether you are a meat eater or vegetarian. Do not use half-and-half or milk since there is carbohydrate in milk or half-and-half and none in heavy cream. You will enjoy the heavy cream more. The reason I put black coffee is so you don't think you can add any Creamora or any cream substitute because such products are loaded with sugar or sugar substitute.

Meat eaters complain that the thirty-day diet plan includes expensive cuts of meats. Remember that this is for just thirty days. After the thirty days you can save all the money you want. Usually you eat out in fast food restaurants or you may even go to expensive restaurants and think nothing of the bill. If you could sacrifice eating out for one month I think that should easily cover the extra cost of the expensive cuts of meats. How much do you spend on your bar bill or the liquor store a month? If you follow my suggestions you will save on junk food, sugar items, desserts, pastries, liquor and many other sugar products. The savings from avoiding these products for a month more than off sets or balances the expensive meats. But of course, you may substitute the expensive cuts of meats with the inexpensive cuts. So don't get all excited when you see an expensive cut of meat on the diet, since you as the *diet authority* may substitute the expensive cut with an inexpensive one. If you substitute carbohydrate, just be sure to stay with the 30 grams a day limit.

30-Day Meat Eaters Rosacea Diet Plan

	Meat Eaters Menu Anyone may Eat as much protein as you want! SUBSTITUTE any PROTEIN with a Protein	Carbohydrate Grams Just Limit your Carbohydrate To 30 Grams per day!
Day One		
breakfast	at wake up—12 oz. glass of water, Sausage and eggs, salt, one cup black coffee or tea, 12 oz glass of water, vitamins	Zero carbs
Break	12 oz glass of water, cheese	5 oz of cheddar—3 grams carbs
Lunch	12 oz glass of water, half avocado with tuna, chicken, or crab with vinegar & oil, chopped hard-boiled egg with fresh salad greens, black olives, tomato (vinegar and oil) one cup black coffee or tea, 12 oz glass of water	half Florida avocado—6.5 grams carbs 1 cup of salad greens—2 grams carbs Half tomato—3 grams carbs
Break	12 oz glass of water, cheese	5 oz of cheddar—3 grams carbs
Supper	12 oz glass of water, Beef tenderloin (or other lean cut) asparagus spears with cheese, fresh green salad (vinegar and oil) tea, 12 oz. glass of water	4 asparagus spears—2.2 grams carbs 5 oz cheese—3 grams carbs 1 cup of salad—2 grams carbs
Day One	Before bed 12 oz glass of water, if you wake up in the night, drink 12 oz glass of water	Total carbohydrate = Less than 30 grams carbs

	Meat Eaters Menu Anyone may Eat as much protein as you want! SUBSTITUTE any PROTEIN with a Protein	Carbohydrate Grams Just Limit your Carbohydrate to 30 grams per day!
Day Two		
breakfast	at wake up—12 oz. glass of water, Bacon [not sugar cured] and eggs, salt one cup black coffee or tea, 12 oz glass of water, vitamins	Zero carbs
Break	12 oz glass of water, cheese	5 oz of cheddar = 3 grams carbs
Lunch	12 oz glass of water, pork chops, cottage cheese fresh green salad (vinegar and oil) with tomato one cup black coffee or tea, 12 oz glass of water	1 cup whole milk cottage cheese— 8 grams carbs 1 cup of salad greens— 2 grams carbs Half tomato—3 grams carbs
Break	12 oz glass of water, cheese (your choice)	5 oz of cheddar—3 grams carbs
Supper	12 oz glass of water, meat loaf (no sugar, syrup, catsup, raisins, carrots in meatloaf) cabbage cole slaw or fresh green salad (vinegar and oil) 12 oz glass of water, tea	Half cup cole slaw w/dressing —4.25 grams carbs or 1 cup of salad greens —2 grams carbs
Day Two	Before bed 12 oz glass of water, if you wake up in the night, drink 12 oz glass of water	Total carbohydrate = Less than 30 grams carbs

Day Three	Meat Eaters Menu Anyone may Eat as much protein as you want! SUBSTITUTE any PROTEIN with a Protein	Carbohydrate Grams Just Limit your Carbohydrate to 30 grams per day!
breakfast	at wake up—12 oz. glass of water, cheese omelet, salt, one cup black coffee or tea 12 oz glass of water, vitamins	5 oz. cheese in omelet—3 grams carbs
break	12 oz glass of water, nuts with celery	1 tablespoon mixed nuts—2 grams carbs 2 stalks celery—3 grams carbs
Lunch	12 oz glass of water, chicken, Cole slaw (no sugar in dressing) or fresh green salad (vinegar and oil) one cup black coffee or tea 12 oz glass of water	Half cup cole slaw w/dressing—4.25 grams carbs or 1 cup of salad greens—2 grams carbs
Break	12 oz glass of water, nuts with celery	1 tablespoon mixed nuts—2 grams carbs 2 stalks celery—3 grams carbs
Supper	12 oz glass of water, meat loaf (no sugar, syrup, catsup, raisins, carrots in meatloaf) cabbage cole slaw, fresh green salad (vinegar and oil) 12 oz glass of water, tea	Half cup cole slaw w/dressing—4.25 grams carbs 1 cup of salad greens—2 grams carbs
Day Three	Before bed 12 oz glass of water, if you wake up in the night, drink 12 oz glass of water	Total carbohydrate = Less than 30 grams carbs

Day Four	Meat Eaters Menu Anyone may Eat as much protein as you want! SUBSTITUTE any PROTEIN with a Protein	Carbohydrate Grams Just Limit your Carbohydrate to 30 grams per day!
breakfast	at wake up—12 oz. glass of water, Bacon [not sugar cured] and eggs, salt, one cup black coffee or tea, 12 oz glass of water, vitamins	Zero carbs
Break	12 oz glass of water, cheese	5 oz cheese—3 grams carbs
Lunch	12 oz glass of water, fish, half avocado and peppers green salad (vinegar and oil) one cup black coffee or tea 12 oz glass of water	Half Calif. Avocado—6.5 grams carbs Half cup green pepper—3 grams carbs 1 cup of salad greens—2 grams carbs
Break	12 oz glass of water, cheese	5 oz cheese—3 grams carbs
Supper	12 oz glass of water, corned beef and cabbage, fresh green salad (vinegar and oil) 12 oz glass of water, tea	1 cup cooked cabbage—6 grams carbs 1 cup of salad greens—2 grams carbs
Day Four	Before bed 12 oz glass of water, if you wake up in the night, drink 12 oz glass of water	Total carbohydrate = Less than 30 grams carbs

Day Five	Meat Eaters Menu Anyone may Eat as much protein as you want! SUBSTITUTE any PROTEIN with a Protein	Carbohydrate Grams Just Limit your Carbohydrate to 30 grams per day!
breakfast	at wake up—12 oz. glass of water, Canadian bacon [not sugar cured] & eggs, salt, one cup black coffee or tea, 12 oz glass of water, vitamins	Trace carbs in Canadian Bacon
Break	12 oz glass of water, cheese and nuts	5 oz cheese—3 grams carbs 2 tablespoons of Mixed nuts— 3.5 grams carbs
Lunch	12 oz glass of water, hamburger patty and cottage cheese fresh green salad (vinegar and oil) one cup black coffee or tea 12 oz glass of water	One cup of whole milk cottage cheese—8 grams carbs 1 cup of salad greens—2 grams carbs
Break	12 oz glass of water, celery with cream cheese and nuts	tablespoons cream cheese— 2 grams carbs 2 stalks celery—3.2 grams carbs 1 tablespoon mixed nuts— 2.3 grams carbs
Supper	12 oz glass of water, chef salad with meat (vinegar and oil) 12 oz glass of water, tea	Chef salad—5 grams carbs estimated
Day Five	Before bed 12 oz glass of water, if you wake up in the night, drink 12 oz glass of water	Total carbohydrate = around 30 grams carbs

	Meat Eaters Menu Anyone may Eat as much protein as you want! SUBSTITUTE any PROTEIN with a Protein	**Carbohydrate Grams** Just Limit your Carbohydrate to 30 grams per day!
Day Six		
breakfast	at wake up—12 oz. glass of water, steak & eggs, salt, one cup black coffee or tea, 12 oz glass of water, vitamins	Zero carbs
Break	12 oz glass of water, cheese and nuts	5 oz cheese—3 grams carbs 2 tablespoons of Mixed nuts— 4.6 grams carbs
Lunch	12 oz glass of water, fish with tofu or spinach fresh green salad (vinegar and oil) one cup black coffee or tea 12 oz glass of water	One cup cooked spinach—6.5 grams carbs 1 cup of salad greens—2 grams carbs
Break	12 oz glass of water, celery with cream cheese and nuts	4 tablespoons cream cheese—2 grams carbs 2 stalks celery—3.2 grams carbs
Supper	12 oz glass of water, cheeseburger patty and eggplant fresh green salad (vinegar and oil) 12 oz glass of water	Half cup eggplant—4.1 grams carbs 1 cup of salad greens—2 grams carbs
Day Six	Before bed 12 oz glass of water, if you wake up in the night, drink 12 oz glass of water	Total carbohydrate = less than 30 grams carbs

Day Seven	**Meat Eaters Menu** Anyone may Eat as much protein as you want! SUBSTITUTE any PROTEIN with a Protein	**Carbohydrate Grams** Just Limit your Carbohydrate to 30 grams per day!
breakfast	at wake up—12 oz. glass of water, tofu or eggs and cottage cheese one cup black coffee or tea, 12 oz glass of water, vitamins	Half cup whole milk cottage cheese—4 grams carbs 2 in. cube tofu—2.9 grams carbs
Break	12 oz glass of water, two hard boiled eggs	zero carbs
Lunch	12 oz glass of water, fish and peppers, broccoli, OR green beans fresh green salad (vinegar and oil) one cup black coffee or tea 12 oz glass of water	Half cup diced peppers— 3 grams carbs Half cup broccoli—4 grams carbs Half cup green snap beans— 3.4 grams carbs 1 cup of salad greens— 2 grams carbs
Break	12 oz glass of water, celery with cream cheese and nuts	2 tablespoons cream cheese— 1 grams carbs 2 stalks celery—3.2 grams carbs 1 tablespoons mixed nuts— 2 grams carbs
Supper	12 oz glass of water, steak and asparagus, salt, fresh green salad (vinegar and oil) 12 oz glass of water	4 asparagus spears—2.2 grams carbs 1 cup of salad greens— 2 grams carbs
Day Seven	Before bed 12 oz glass of water, if you wake up in the night, drink 12 oz glass of water	Total carbohydrate = less than 30 grams carbs

Day Eight	Meat Eaters Menu Anyone may Eat as much protein as you want! SUBSTITUTE any PROTEIN with a Protein	Carbohydrate Grams Just Limit your Carbohydrate to 30 grams per day!
breakfast	at wake up—12 oz. glass of water, cheese omelet with celery and peppers one cup black coffee or tea 12 oz glass of water, vitamins	2 oz cheese—.1.2 grams carbs 1 stalk celery—1.6 grams carbs Quarter cup green peppers— 2.5 grams carbs
Break	12 oz glass of water, cheese and nuts	2 oz cheese—1.2 grams carbs One and half tablespoons of mixed nuts—3.5 grams carbs
Lunch	12 oz glass of water, steak and eggs fresh green salad (vinegar and oil) one cup black coffee or tea 12 oz glass of water	1 cup of salad greens— 2 grams carbs
Break	12 oz glass of water, celery with cream cheese and nuts	2 tablespoons cream cheese— 1 grams carbs 2 stalks celery—3.2 grams carbs One and half tablespoons of mixed nuts—3.5 grams carbs
Supper	12 oz glass of water, fish with cucumbers, mushrooms, peppers fresh green salad (vinegar and oil) 12 oz glass of water	Half cucumber—1.8 grams carbs Half cup mushrooms—2.6 grams carbs Half cup green pepper—3.6 grams carbs 1 cup of salad greens—2 grams carbs

| Day Eight | Before bed 12 oz glass of water, if you wake up in the night, drink 12 oz glass of water | Total carbohydrate = around 30 grams carbs |

Day Nine	Meat Eaters Menu Anyone may Eat as much protein as you want! SUBSTITUTE any PROTEIN with a Protein	Carbohydrate Grams Just Limit your Carbohydrate to 30 grams per day!
breakfast	at wake up—12 oz. glass of water, steak and eggs, salt, one cup black coffee or tea, 12 oz glass of water, vitamins	zero carbs
Break	12 oz glass of water, cheese and nuts 3 oz cheese	5 oz cheese—3 grams carbs Three tablespoons of mixed nuts— 7 grams carbs
Lunch	12 oz glass of water, fish and green peppers, fresh green salad (vinegar and oil) one cup black coffee or tea 12 oz glass of water	One pepper—7.2 grams carbs 1 cup of salad greens— 2 grams carbs
Break	12 oz glass of water, two hard boiled eggs, nuts	One and half tablespoons of mixed nuts—3.5 grams carbs
Supper	12 oz glass of water, chef salad with meat (vinegar and oil) 12 oz glass of water, tea	chef salad—5 grams carbs estimated
Day Nine	Before bed 12 oz glass of water, if you wake up in the night, drink 12 oz glass of water	Total carbohydrate = less than 30 grams carbs

Day Ten	Meat Eaters Menu Anyone may Eat as much protein as you want! SUBSTITUTE any PROTEIN with a Protein	Carbohydrate Grams Just Limit your Carbohydrate to 30 grams per day!
breakfast	at wake up—12 oz. glass of water, sausage and eggs one cup black coffee or tea, 12 oz glass of water, vitamins	zero carbs
Break	12 oz glass of water, cheese and nuts	3 oz cheese—1.8 grams carbs One and half tablespoons of mixed nuts—3.5 grams carbs
Lunch	12 oz glass of water, cheeseburger patty and cottage cheese fresh green salad (vinegar and oil) one cup black coffee or tea 12 oz glass of water	2 oz cheese—1.2 grams carbs 1 cup of salad greens—2 grams carbs
Break	12 oz glass of water, celery with cream cheese and nuts	2 stalks celery—3.2 grams carbs 2 tablespoons cream cheese— 2 grams carbs 3 tablespoons mixed nuts—7 grams carbs
Supper	12 oz glass of water, steak with mushrooms, zucchini, spinach fresh green salad (vinegar and oil) 12 oz glass of water	Half cup mushrooms—1.5 grams carbs Half cup zucchini—2.6 grams carbs 1 cup raw spinach—2.4 grams carbs
Day Ten	Before bed 12 oz glass of water, if you wake up in the night, drink 12 oz glass of water	Total carbohydrate = less than 30 grams carbs

Day Eleven	Meat Eaters Menu Anyone may Eat as much protein as you want! SUBSTITUTE any PROTEIN with a Protein	Carbohydrate Grams Just Limit your Carbohydrate to 30 grams per day!
breakfast	at wake up—12 oz. glass of water, cheese omelet with cottage cheese one cup black coffee or tea, 12 oz glass of water, vitamins	3 oz cheese—1.2 grams carbs Half cup whole milk cottage cheese— 4 grams carbs
Break	12 oz glass of water, celery with cream cheese and nuts	3 stalks celery—4.8 grams carbs 3 tablespoons cream cheese— 1.5 grams carbs One and half tablespoons of mixed nuts—3.5 grams carbs
Lunch	12 oz glass of water, pork chops and green beans, fresh green salad (vinegar and oil), one cup black coffee or tea, 12 oz glass of water	Half cup snap green beans— 3.4 grams carb 1 cup of salad greens— 2 grams carbs
Break	12 oz glass of water, two hard boiled eggs	zero carbs
Supper	12 oz glass of water, chicken with spinach, fresh green salad (vinegar and oil) 12 oz glass of water, tea	One cup cooked spinach— 6.5 grams carbs 1 cup of salad greens— 2 grams carbs
Day Eleven	Before bed 12 oz glass of water, if you wake up in the night, drink 12 oz glass of water	Total carbohydrate = less than 30 grams carbs

Day Twelve	Meat Eaters Menu Anyone may Eat as much protein as you want! SUBSTITUTE any PROTEIN with a Protein	Carbohydrate Grams Just Limit your Carbohydrate to 30 grams per day!
breakfast	at wake up—12 oz. glass of water, bacon [not sugar cured] and eggs, salt, one cup black coffee or tea, 12 oz glass of water, vitamins	zero carbs
Break	12 oz glass of water, celery with almond butter	2 stalks celery—3.2 grams carbs Quarter oz almond butter— 3.6 grams carbs
Lunch	12 oz glass of water, salmon with broccoli, fresh green salad (vinegar and oil) one cup black coffee or tea 12 oz glass of water	Half cup broccoli—4.25 grams/carb 1 cup of salad greens— 2 grams carbs
Break	12 oz glass of water, celery with cream cheese and nuts	3 stalks celery—4.8 grams carbs 3 tablespoons cream cheese— 1.5 grams carbs One and half tablespoons of mixed nuts—3.5 grams carbs
Supper	12 oz glass of water, Pork loin with asparagus/melted cheese fresh green salad (vinegar and oil) 12 oz glass of water, tea	1 oz cheese—.6 gram/carb 8 asparagus spears— 4.4 grams carbs 1 cup of salad greens— 2 grams carbs
Day Twelve	Before bed 12 oz glass of water, if you wake up in the night, drink 12 oz glass of water	Total carbohydrate = less than 30 grams carbs

Day Thirteen	Meat Eaters Menu Anyone may Eat as much protein as you want! SUBSTITUTE any PROTEIN with a Protein	Carbohydrate Grams Just Limit your Carbohydrate to 30 grams per day!
breakfast	at wake up—12 oz. glass of water, eggs and sausage, salt, one cup black coffee or tea, 12 oz glass of water, vitamins	zero carbs
Break	12 oz glass of water, celery with cream cheese and nuts	2 stalks celery—3.2 grams carbs 3 tablespoons cream cheese— 1.5 grams carbs One and half tablespoons of mixed nuts—3.5 grams carbs
Lunch	12 oz glass of water, steak with eggplant, fresh green salad (vinegar and oil) one cup black coffee or tea 12 oz glass of water	Half cup eggplant—4.1 grams carb 1 cup of salad greens—2 grams carbs
Break	12 oz glass of water, cheese and nuts	3 oz cheese—1.8 grams carbs One and half tablespoons of mixed nuts—3.5 grams carbs
Supper	12 oz glass of water, prime roast beef with mushrooms and green beans fresh green salad (vinegar and oil) 12 oz glass of water, tea	Half cup mushrooms—2.5 gram carb Half cup snap green beans— 3.4 grams carbs 1 cup of salad greens—2 grams carbs
Day Thirteen	Before bed 12 oz glass of water, if you wake up in the night, drink 12 oz glass of water	Total carbohydrate = less than 30 grams carbs

Day Fourteen	Meat Eaters Menu Anyone may Eat as much protein as you want! SUBSTITUTE any PROTEIN with a Protein	Carbohydrate Grams Just Limit your Carbohydrate to 30 grams per day!
breakfast	at wake up—12 oz. glass of water, cheese omelet with celery and peppers. one cup black coffee or tea, 12 oz glass of water, vitamins	1 oz. cheese—.6 grams carbs 1 stalk celery—1.6 grams carbs Half cup green pepper—3.4 grams carbs
Break	12 oz glass of water, nuts	3 tablespoons of mixed nuts—7 grams carbs
Lunch	12 oz glass of water, cheeseburger patty with mushrooms fresh green salad (vinegar and oil) one cup black coffee or tea 12 oz glass of water	Half cup eggplant—4.1 grams carb 1 cup of salad greens—2 grams carbs
Break	12 oz glass of water, celery with cream cheese	3 stalks celery—4.8 grams carbs 3 tablespoons cream cheese—1.5 grams carbs
Supper	12 oz glass of water, fillet mignon and mushrooms fresh green salad (vinegar and oil) 12 oz glass of water, tea	Half cup mushrooms—2.5 gram carb 1 cup of salad greens—2 grams carbs
Day Fourteen	Before bed 12 oz glass of water, if you wake up in the night, drink 12 oz glass of water	Total carbohydrate = less than 30 grams carbs

Day Fifteen	Meat Eaters Menu Anyone may Eat as much protein as you want! SUBSTITUTE any PROTEIN with a Protein	Carbohydrate Grams Just Limit your Carbohydrate to 30 grams per day!
breakfast	at wake up—12 oz. glass of water, Ham and eggs, one cup black coffee, or tea, 12 oz glass of water, vitamins	zero carbs
Break	12 oz glass of water, nuts	3 tablespoons of mixed nuts— 7 grams carbs
Lunch	12 oz glass of water, fish or seafood [no batter] spinach, fresh green salad with vinegar and oil, one cup black coffee or tea 12 oz glass of water	1 cup spinach—6.5 grams carb 1 cup of salad greens— 2 grams carbs
Break	12 oz glass of water, celery with cream cheese	3 stalks celery—4.8 grams carbs 3 tablespoons cream cheese— 1.5 grams carbs
Supper	12 oz glass of water, Pork or Lamb, scallions, peppers, and fresh lettuce, grape tomatoes with vinegar and oil 12 oz glass of water, tea	2 tablespoons scallions— 2 grams carbs 1 cup of salad greens— 2 grams carbs 5 grape tomatoes— 3 grams carbs
Day Fifteen	Before bed 12 oz glass of water, if you wake up in the night, drink 12 oz glass of water	Total carbohydrate = less than 30 grams carbs

Day Sixteen	Meat Eaters Menu Anyone may Eat as much protein as you want! SUBSTITUTE any PROTEIN with a Protein	Carbohydrate Grams Just Limit your Carbohydrate to 30 grams per day!
breakfast	at wake up—12 oz. glass of water, Steak and eggs, salt, one cup black coffee, or tea 12 oz glass of water, vitamins	zero carbs
Break	12 oz glass of water, nuts	3 tablespoons of mixed nuts— 7 grams carbs
Lunch	12 oz glass of water, cheeseburger patty with mushrooms fresh green salad (vinegar and oil) one cup black coffee or tea 12 oz glass of water	1 oz cheese—.6 grams carb 1 cup of salad greens—2 grams carbs
Break	12 oz glass of water, two hard boiled eggs	zero carbs
Supper	12 oz glass of water, fish or seafood [no batter], collard greens, fresh green salad with vinegar and oil, one cup black coffee or tea 12 oz glass of water	1 cup collard greens—9.8 grams carbs 1 cup of salad greens—2 grams carbs 5 grape tomatoes—3 grams carbs
Day Sixteen	Before bed 12 oz glass of water, if you wake up in the night, drink 12 oz glass of water	Total carbohydrate = less than 30 grams carbs

	Meat Eaters Menu Anyone may Eat as much protein as you want! SUBSTITUTE any PROTEIN with a Protein	Carbohydrate Grams Just Limit your Carbohydrate to 30 grams per day!
Day Seventeen		
breakfast	at wake up—12 oz. glass of water, bacon [not sugar cured] and eggs with one cup black coffee, or tea, 12 oz glass of water, vitamins	zero carbs
Break	12 oz glass of water, nuts	3 tablespoons of mixed nuts—7 grams carbs
Lunch	12 oz glass of water, salmon with salsa, asparagus spears & butter fresh green salad (vinegar and oil) one cup black coffee or tea 12 oz glass of water	2 tablespoons salsa—2.5 grams carbs 4 asparagus spears—2.2 grams carbs 1 cup of salad greens—2 grams carbs
Break	12 oz glass of water, celery with cream cheese	2 stalks celery—3.2 grams carbs 2 tablespoons cream cheese—1 grams carbs
Supper	12 oz glass of water, baked ham [salt cured, not sugar cured] and collard greens fresh green salad (vinegar and oil) 12 oz glass of water, tea	1 cup collard greens—9.8 grams carbs 1 cup of salad greens—2 grams carbs
Day Seventeen	Before bed 12 oz glass of water, if you wake up in the night, drink 12 oz glass of water	Total carbohydrate = less than 30 grams carbs

Day Eighteen	**Meat Eaters Menu** Anyone may Eat as much protein as you want! SUBSTITUTE any PROTEIN with a Protein	**Carbohydrate Grams** Just Limit your Carbohydrate to 30 grams per day!
breakfast	at wake up—12 oz. glass of water, Spanish omelet, salt, one cup black coffee, or tea, 12 oz glass of water, vitamins	Half cup green peppers—3.6 grams carbs Half tomato—3 grams carbs Quarter cup onions—3.7 grams carbs 1 oz cheese—.6 gram/carb
Break	12 oz glass of water, celery	3 celery stalks—4.8 grams carbs
Lunch	12 oz glass of water, chicken, turnip, fresh green salad with vinegar and oil, one cup black coffee or tea 12 oz glass of water	Half turnip—4.3 grams carbs 1 cup of salad greens—2 grams carbs
Break	12 oz glass of water, two hard boiled eggs	zero carbs
Supper	12 oz glass of water, Pork tenderloin, spinach, olives, scallions, fresh lettuce salad, vinegar and oil 12 oz glass of water, tea 12 oz glass of water, tea	Half cup spinach—3.25 grams carbs 4 black olives—1 grams carbs 2 tablespoons scallions—1 gram carb 1 cup of salad greens—2 grams carbs
Day Eighteen	Before bed 12 oz glass of water, if you wake up in the night, drink 12 oz glass of water	Total carbohydrate = less than 30 grams carbs

	Meat Eaters Menu Anyone may Eat as much protein as you want! SUBSTITUTE any PROTEIN with a Protein	Carbohydrate Grams Just Limit your Carbohydrate to 30 grams per day!
Day Nineteen		
breakfast	at wake up—12 oz. glass of water, steak and eggs, salt, one cup black coffee, or tea 12 oz glass of water, vitamins	zero carbs
Break	12 oz glass of water, celery	2 stalks celery—3.2 grams carbs
Lunch	12 oz glass of water, lamb chops, cucumbers, tomato, fresh green salad (vinegar and oil) one cup black coffee or tea 12 oz glass of water	Half cucumber—1.8 grams carbs 1 tomato—5.8 grams carbs, 1 cup of salad greens— 2 grams carbs
Break	12 oz glass of water, two hard boiled eggs	zero carbs
Supper	12 oz glass of water, Pork roast, wild rice, mushrooms, fresh green salad (vinegar and oil) 12 oz glass of water	Half cup wild rice—11 grams carbs Half cup mushrooms—1.6 gram carb 1 cup of salad greens— 2 grams carbs
Day Nineteen	Before bed 12 oz glass of water, if you wake up in the night, drink 12 oz glass of water	Total carbohydrate = less than 30 grams carbs

Day Twenty	Meat Eaters Menu Anyone may Eat as much protein as you want! SUBSTITUTE any PROTEIN with a Protein	Carbohydrate Grams Just Limit your Carbohydrate to 30 grams per day!
breakfast	at wake up—12 oz. glass of water, cottage cheese and eggs one cup black coffee, or tea, 12 oz glass of water, vitamins	half cup cottage cheese— 4 grams carbs
Break	12 oz glass of water, nuts	3 tablespoons of mixed nuts— 7 grams carbs
Lunch	12 oz glass of water, hamburger patty with mushrooms fresh green salad with vinegar and oil, one cup black coffee or tea 12 oz glass of water	Half cup mushrooms— 1.6 grams carbs 1 cup of salad greens—2 grams carbs
Break	12 oz glass of water, celery and cream cheese	2 stalks celery—3.2 grams carbs 2 tablespoons cream cheese— 1 grams carbs
Supper	12 oz glass of water, Roast beef, broccoli or Brussels sprouts fresh lettuce, with vinegar and oil 12 oz glass of water, tea	Half cup broccoli—4.25 grams carbs Half cup Brussels sprouts— 5 grams carbs 1 cup of salad greens— 2 grams carbs
Day Twenty	Before bed 12 oz glass of water, if you wake up in the night, drink 12 oz glass of water	Total carbohydrate = less than 30 grams carbs

Day Twenty One	Meat Eaters Menu Anyone may Eat as much protein as you want! SUBSTITUTE any PROTEIN with a Protein	Carbohydrate Grams Just Limit your Carbohydrate to 30 grams per day!
breakfast	at wake up—12 oz. glass of water, Sausage, and eggs salt, one cup black coffee, or tea, 12 oz glass of water, vitamins	half cup cottage cheese— 4 grams carbs
Break	12 oz glass of water, cheese	5 oz cheese—3 grams carbs
Lunch	12 oz glass of water, fish or seafood, cole slaw, fresh salad greens, black olives, tomato (vinegar and oil) one cup black coffee or tea 12 oz glass of water	Half cup cole slaw— 4.25 grams carbs 4 black olives—1 grams carbs 1 cup of salad greens— 2 grams carbs
Break	12 oz glass of water, cheese	5 oz cheese—3 grams carbs
Supper	12 oz glass of water, Beef tenderloin (or other lean cut) asparagus spears with cheese fresh green salad (vinegar and oil) 12 oz glass of water, tea	8 asparagus spears— 4.4 grams carbs grams carbs 5 oz cheese—5 grams carbs 1 cup of salad greens— 2 grams carbs
Day Twenty One	Before bed 12 oz glass of water, if you wake up in the night, drink 12 oz glass of water	Total carbohydrate = less than 30 grams carbs

Day Twenty Two	**Meat Eaters Menu** Anyone may Eat as much protein as you want! SUBSTITUTE any PROTEIN with a Protein	**Carbohydrate Grams** Just Limit your Carbohydrate to 30 grams per day!
breakfast	at wake up—12 oz. glass of water, Bacon [not sugar cured] and eggs [little salt/pepper] one cup black coffee, or tea, 12 oz glass of water, vitamins	zero carbohydrate
Break	12 oz glass of water, two hard boiled eggs	Break zero carbohydrate
Lunch	12 oz glass of water, shish kebab green salad (vinegar and oil) one cup black coffee or tea 12 oz glass of water	shish kabob vegetables— 20 grams carbs estimated 1 cup of salad greens— 2 grams carbs
Break	12 oz glass of water, tofu	zero carbohydrate
Supper	12 oz glass of water, corned beef and cabbage, fresh green salad (vinegar and oil) 12 oz glass of water, tea	1 cup cabbage—6.2 grams carbs grams carbs 1 cup of salad greens— 2 grams carbs
Day Twenty Two	Before bed 12 oz glass of water, if you wake up in the night, drink 12 oz glass of water	Total carbohydrate = less than 30 grams carbs

Day Twenty Three	**Meat Eaters Menu** Anyone may Eat as much protein as you want! SUBSTITUTE any PROTEIN with a Protein	**Carbohydrate Grams** Just Limit your Carbohydrate to 30 grams per day!
breakfast	at wake up—12 oz. glass of water, cheese omelet with celery and peppers one cup black coffee, or tea, 12 oz glass of water, vitamins	3 oz cheese—1.8 grams carbs 1 stalk of celery—1.6 grams carbs Quarter cup green peppers— 1.8 grams carbs
Break	12 oz glass of water, nuts	3 tablespoons mixed nuts— 7 grams carbs
Lunch	12 oz glass of water, steak and eggs, salt, fresh green salad (vinegar and oil) one cup black coffee or tea 12 oz glass of water	1 cup of salad greens— 2 grams carbs
Break	12 oz glass of water, nuts	3 tablespoons mixed nuts— 7 grams carbs
Supper	12 oz glass of water, fish with cucumbers, mushrooms, peppers fresh green salad (vinegar and oil) 12 oz glass of water, tea	Half cucumber—1.8 grams carbs Half cup mushrooms— 1.6 grams carbs Half pepper—3.6 grams carbs 1 cup of salad greens— 2 grams carbs
Day Twenty Three	Before bed 12 oz glass of water, if you wake up in the night, drink 12 oz glass of water,	Total carbohydrate = less than 30 grams carbs

Day Twenty Four	Meat Eaters Menu Anyone may Eat as much protein as you want! SUBSTITUTE any PROTEIN with a Protein	Carbohydrate Grams Just Limit your Carbohydrate to 30 grams per day!
breakfast	at wake up—12 oz. glass of water, Bacon [not sugar cured] and eggs, salt, one cup black coffee, or tea, 12 oz glass of water, vitamins	zero carbs
Break	12 oz glass of water, cheese	2 oz cheese—1.2 grams carbs
Lunch	12 oz glass of water, pork chops, cottage cheese, fresh green salad (vinegar and oil) one cup black coffee or tea 12 oz glass of water,	1 cup cottage cheese—8 grams carbs 1 cup of salad greens—2 grams carbs
Break	12 oz glass of water, nuts	3 tablespoons mixed nuts—7 grams carbs
Supper	12 oz glass of water, baked ham, collard greens, cabbage coleslaw or fresh green salad (vinegar and oil) 12 oz glass of water, tea	Half cup collard greens—4.9 grams carbs Half cup cole slaw—4.25 grams carbs 1 cup of salad greens—2 grams carbs
Day Twenty Four	Before bed 12 oz glass of water, if you wake up in the night, drink 12 oz glass of water,	Total carbohydrate = less than 30 grams carbs

Day Twenty Five	Meat Eaters Menu Anyone may Eat as much protein as you want! SUBSTITUTE any PROTEIN with a Protein	Carbohydrate Grams Just Limit your Carbohydrate to 30 grams per day!
breakfast	at wake up—12 oz. glass of water, eggs and sausage, salt, one cup black coffee, or tea, 12 oz glass of water, vitamins	zero carbs
Break	12 oz glass of water, celery with cream cheese and nuts	3 stalks celery—4.8 grams carbs 3 tablespoons cream cheese—1.5 grams carbs One and half tablespoons of mixed nuts—3.5 grams carbs
Lunch	12 oz glass of water, steak with eggs fresh green salad (vinegar and oil) one cup black coffee or tea 12 oz glass of water,	1 cup of salad greens—2 grams carbs
Break	12 oz glass of water, nuts	3 tablespoons mixed nuts—7 grams carbs
Supper	12 oz glass of water, prime roast beef with mushrooms and snap green, fresh green salad (vinegar and oil) 12 oz glass of water, tea	Half cup snap greens—3.4 grams carbs Half cup mushrooms—1.6 grams carbs 1 cup of salad greens—2 grams carbs
Day Twenty Five	Before bed 12 oz glass of water, if you wake up in the night, drink 12 oz glass of water	Total carbohydrate = less than 30 grams carbs

Day Twenty Six	**Meat Eaters Menu** Anyone may Eat as much protein as you want! SUBSTITUTE any PROTEIN with a Protein	**Carbohydrate Grams** Just Limit your Carbohydrate to 30 grams per day!
breakfast	at wake up—12 oz. glass of water, cheese omelet, one cup black coffee, or tea, 12 oz glass of water, vitamins	3 Oz cheese—1.8 grams carbs
Break	12-oz glass of water, nuts with celery	3 stalks celery—4.8 grams carbs One and half tablespoons of mixed nuts—3.5 grams carbs
Lunch	12 oz glass of water, chicken, Cole slaw (no sugar in dressing) fresh green salad (vinegar and oil) one cup black coffee or tea 12 oz glass of water	Half cup cole slaw— 4.25 grams carbs 1 cup of salad greens— 2 grams carbs
Break	12 oz glass of water, nuts	2 tablespoons mixed nuts— 4.6 grams carbs
Supper	12 oz glass of water, Sirloin steak, mushrooms, asparagus spears & butter green salad (vinegar and oil) 12 oz glass of water	8 asparagus spears—4.4 grams carbs Half cup mushrooms— 1.6 grams carbs 1 cup of salad greens— 2 grams carbs
Day Twenty Six	Before bed 12 oz glass of water, if you wake up in the night, drink 12 oz glass of water	Total carbohydrate = less than 30 grams carbs

Day Twenty Seven	Meat Eaters Menu Anyone may Eat as much protein as you want! SUBSTITUTE any PROTEIN with a Protein	Carbohydrate Grams Just Limit your Carbohydrate to 30 grams per day!
breakfast	at wake up—12 oz. glass of water, Canadian bacon [not sugar cured] & eggs one cup black coffee, or tea, 12 oz glass of water, vitamins	zero carbs
Break	12 oz glass of water, cheese and nuts	3 Oz cheese—1.8 grams carbs One and half tablespoons of mixed nuts—3.5 grams carbs
Lunch	12 oz glass of water, chicken, Cole slaw (no sugar in dressing) fresh green salad (vinegar and oil) one cup black coffee or tea 12 oz glass of water	Half cup cole slaw—4.25 grams carbs 1 cup of salad greens—2 grams carbs
Break	12 oz glass of water, celery with cream cheese and nuts	3 stalks celery—4.8 grams carbs 3 tablespoons cream cheese—1.5 grams carbs One and half tablespoons of mixed nuts—3.5 grams carbs
Supper	12 oz glass of water, chef salad with meat (vinegar and oil) 12 oz glass of water, tea	chef salad approximately 7 grams carbs
Day Twenty Seven	Before bed 12 oz glass of water, if you wake up in the night, drink 12 oz glass of water	Total carbohydrate = less than 30 grams carbs

Day Twenty Eight	**Meat Eaters Menu** Anyone may Eat as much protein as you want! SUBSTITUTE any PROTEIN with a Protein	**Carbohydrate Grams** Just Limit your Carbohydrate to 30 grams per day!
breakfast	at wake up—12 oz. glass of water, bacon [not sugar cured] and eggs, salt, one cup black coffee, or tea, 12 oz glass of water, vitamins	zero carbs
Break	12 oz glass of water, two hard boiled eggs	zero carbs
Lunch	12 oz glass of water, salmon with broccoli, fresh green salad (vinegar and oil) one cup black coffee or tea 12 oz glass of water	1 cup cole broccoli—7 grams carbs 1 cup of salad greens—2 grams carbs
Break	12 oz glass of water, celery with cream cheese and nuts	3 stalks celery—4.8 grams carbs 3 tablespoons cream cheese— 1.5 grams carbs One and half tablespoons of mixed nuts—3.5 grams carbs
Supper	12 oz glass of water, Pork loin with asparagus with melted cheese, fresh green salad (vinegar and oil) 12 oz glass of water, tea	8 spears asparagus—4.4 grams carbs 3 oz cheese—1.8 grams carbs 1 cup of salad greens— 2 grams carbs
Day Twenty Eight	Before bed 12 oz glass of water, if you wake up in the night, drink 12 oz glass of water	Total carbohydrate = less than 30 grams carbs

Day Twenty Nine	Meat Eaters Menu Anyone may Eat as much protein as you want! SUBSTITUTE any PROTEIN with a Protein	Carbohydrate Grams Just Limit your Carbohydrate to 30 grams per day!
breakfast	at wake up—12 oz. glass of water, tofu or eggs and cottage cheese one cup black coffee or tea, 12 oz glass of water, vitamins	zero carbs
Break	12 oz glass of water, two hard boiled eggs	zero carbs
Lunch	12 oz glass of water, fish and peppers, broccoli, fresh green salad (vinegar and oil), one cup black coffee or tea 12 oz glass of water	1 cup broccoli—7 grams carbs Half cup peppers—3.6 grams carbs 1 cup of salad greens—2 grams carbs
Break	12 oz glass of water, celery with cream cheese and nuts	3 stalks celery—4.8 grams carbs 3 tablespoons cream cheese— 1.5 grams carbs One and half tablespoons of mixed nuts—3.5 grams carbs
Supper	12 oz glass of water, steak and asparagus, fresh green salad (vinegar and oil) 12 oz glass of water, tea	8 spears asparagus—4.4 grams carbs 1 cup of salad greens—2 grams carbs
Day Twenty Nine	Before bed 12 oz glass of water, if you wake up in the night, drink 12 oz glass of water	Total carbohydrate = less than 30 grams carbs

Day Thirty	**Meat Eaters Menu** Anyone may Eat as much protein as you want! SUBSTITUTE any PROTEIN with a Protein	**Carbohydrate Grams** Just Limit your Carbohydrate to 30 grams per day!
breakfast	at wake up—12 oz. glass of water, steak and eggs, salt, one cup black coffee, or tea, 12 oz glass of water, vitamin	zero carbs
Break	12 oz glass of water, two hard boiled eggs	zero carbs
Lunch	12 oz glass of water, lamb chops, cucumbers, tomato, mushrooms fresh green salad (vinegar and oil) one cup black coffee or tea 12 oz glass of water	Half cup cucumbers— 1.8 grams carbs Half cup mushrooms— 1.5 grams carbs Half tomato—2.9 grams carbs 1 cup of salad greens— 2 grams carbs
Break	12 oz glass of water, celery with cream cheese	2 stalks celery—3.2 grams carbs 2 tablespoons cream cheese— 1 grams carbs
Supper	12 oz glass of water, Pork roast, wild rice, mushrooms fresh green salad (vinegar and oil) 12 oz glass of water, tea	Third cup wild rice—14 grams carbs Half cup mushrooms— 1.5 grams carbs 1 cup of salad greens— 2 grams carbs
Day Thirty	Before bed 12 oz glass of water, if you wake up in the night, drink 12 oz glass of water	Total carbohydrate = less than 30 grams carbs

Vegetarians

Vegetarians have been eating a high carbohydrate diet, so this will be difficult but not impossible. The advantage you have as a vegetarian is you have demonstrated your will power by being a vegetarian. The key is to up your protein intake by eating vegetables high in protein, substituting all simple carbohydrate for non-starchy complex carbohydrate, avoiding fruits high in sugar and most important, any type SUGAR! What I have found is vegetarians eat a lot of fruit and sugar! Vegetarians with will power can modify the *Rosacea Diet* by eating more protein and reducing carbohydrate to 30 grams a day, a daunting task, but not impossible.

Why would you even try this diet since you have already chosen to be a vegetarian? Obviously you are a rosacean and wondered what all the hullabaloo was with the *Rosacea Diet* and you saw it was vegetarian friendly. Right? I have found that vegetarians are usually not obese. But if you have been eating tons of sugar and starches you may have a weight problem and this vegetarian diet will prove to you that you can lose weight as well. The *Rosacea Diet* will prove also that you can feel healthier if you up your protein. Once you have proven this to yourself, you can then decide what to do about your protein deficiency. The *30-Day Vegetarian Diet Plan* is simply to prove to yourself that you need more protein to control your rosacea. After the thirty days you can return to your previous vegetarian diet and see the difference. You will decide from this experiment whether or not you need more protein in your diet when your rosacea is controlled. The only way to know is try it. It is only thirty days of your life.

If you are an orthodox vegetarian [a vegan who avoids all products of animal origin, including milk and eggs] the highest source of protein in the vegetable world is soy, and eating soy products for a month isn't a feast, but also isn't a famine. Consider it a soy fast! There are a number of soy products on the market now that substitute meat and cheese which you no doubt are aware of. If you know of another source of vegetable in higher protein power than soy let me know. Depending on your orthodox vegetarian beliefs, you may eat eggs and cheese for thirty days along with the soy products. However, if you are a liberal vegetarian (an ovo-lacto vegetarian allowing eggs or dairy or a vegetarian allowing fowl, fish or shellfish) this makes the task easier to reduce your carbohydrate to 30 grams a day and have more variety in protein. If you are an orthodox vegetarian [vegan], is it possible to change your beliefs for just thirty days and be a liberal vegetarian allowing fowl, fish, or shellfish for the sake a clearer face? It is just for thirty days! If this is not possible set your mind on a soy fast for thirty days! If you can eat eggs, consider an egg fast for thirty days! Orthodox vegetarians should either substitute soy or eggs for the PROTEIN suggested in the thirty-day diet plan or simply add them to the menu. You can eat as many eggs or as much protein powder as you want as long as the **protein powder has zero carbohydrate**. After the thirty days, you can eat whatever you want. Here are some suggestions on protein powder:

Trader Joe's Soy Protein Powder uses a "soy isolate," the chemistry used to isolate the soy that may have health ramifications for some, so I have included here three organic alternatives:

Iso-Rich Soy has 0 grams of sugar per 2 rounded tablespoons (28 g) of powder with water
Fermented Soy Essence™ has 2 grams of sugar per 2 rounded tablespoons (28 g) with water
Iso-Rich Soy Greens™ has 0 grams of sugar has per 2 tablespoons (31 g) of powder with water

The above three products are available at the following url:

http://www.jarrow.com

Remember to use just water or any liquid with zero carbohydrate such as cream with your protein powder. NO JUICE! Juice has too much carbohydrate.

Liberal vegetarians may substitute the vegetables suggested in the thirty-day diet plan with soy products that contain no sugar such as tofu, protein powder without any carbohydrate or sugar substitutes, fowl, fish, or shellfish, if allowed. So liberal vegetarians have more variety during the thirty days. For carbohydrate you may use dairy products (without fruit or sugar) and the vegetables mentioned at the end of this chapter. Avoid fruits and vegetables that are high in sugar content such as, potatoes (any color), white rice, corn, popcorn, cornbread, cornmeal, carrots, beets, white flour, and pasta which are all high in carbohydrate. Eat whole grains without sugar, honey, or any other sweetener during this thirty-day diet plan [ABSOLUTELY NO WHITE FLOUR] and no sugar substitutes. But remember no matter what carbohydrate you eat, the TOTAL NUMBER OF GRAMS PER DAY SHOULD BE LESS THAN 30 GRAMS! **You have the same carbohydrate limit as meat eaters**. For example, if you choose to eat one slice of whole wheat bread, which contains 11 grams of carbohydrate, you only have 19 grams left of carbohydrate to eat for the whole day! One cup of milk contains 11 grams of carbs. I know this is not easy, but vegetarians who wish to control their rosacea with their diet must have will power. If you can, avoid grains entirely for thirty days.

Avoid raisins, bananas, all fruits high in carbohydrate, fruit juices, parsnips, honey, carrots, corn/cornflakes, corn products, millet, beets, white rice, pasta, plain crackers, all types of white flour, any potatoes (any color), oatmeal or WHITE breads JUST FOR THIRTY DAYS. It will be extremely difficult to only eat 30 grams of carbohydrate a day, but it can be done by an orthodox vegetarian with will power. For example, two scoops (28 grams) of Trader Joe's Soy Protein Powder have 1 gram of fat and 23 grams of protein with ZERO carbohydrate. That gives you an idea of how to do it. Depending on what type of vegetarian you are, substitute the meats in the *Rosacea Diet* with eggs, cheese, fish, fowl, shellfish, or soy products. An excellent source to count carbohydrate grams is found in the chapter on *Reading the Nutrition Label.*

Vegans usually are aware of the lack of vitamin B12 in the their diet. B12 is generally assumed to be found only in animal products. B12 is difficult to obtain from plants but does occur in some fermented plant foods, such as tempeh, miso, etc. A B12 supplement can help assure adequate amounts in the vegan diet. B12 occurs as a molecule with an atom of cobalt at its center but does not technically come from animals or plants since microorganisms such as bacteria and algae make it. These are found in and on the foods we eat. The bacteria in the live-stock's digestive system spread the B12 vitamin throughout the flesh and milk. If you are a vegetarian who eats eggs and dairy products you will get B12 in your diet. If you are a vegan, you should think about B12 supplements. More information on B12 can be found at this url >

http://www.earthsave.bc.ca/materials/articles/health/b12.html

Soy is the only known plant with all nine essential amino acids and is an excellent source of protein for vegans (see the chapters, Protein and Protein Synthesis). For thirty days vegetarians should eat a high protein diet to lose control their rosacea. If after thirty days you notice a differ-ence you may want to seriously consider whether your current diet is protein deficient and decide what to do about it. The 30-Day Diet Plan for Vegetarians is for vegans. If you can add protein such as fish, fowl, eggs, or dairy then you have additional sources in whatever amounts you want since these sources of protein rarely have any carbohydrate.

Vegetarians may substitute any of the following:

Fish or Shell Fish (if allowed)
Fowl—i.e., chicken or Turkey (if allowed)
Eggs
Soy Products (soy milk, cereals with no sugar, soy burgers, soy links, etc., note any carbohydrate in the product and add into the 30 grams a day limit)
Soy Protein Powder with ZERO carbohydrate or sugar/sugar substitutes
Protein Powder (egg or other source acceptable to you) with no sugar/sugar substitutes that contains zero carbohydrate on the Nutrition Facts Label
Tofu, Tempeh, Miso
Nonstarchy vegetables low in carbohydrate
asparagus, bamboo shoots, bean sprouts, bok choy, broccoli, cabbage, chinese cabbage, cauliflower, celery, collards, cucumber, dandelion greens, egg plant, endive, escarole, garlic, green pepper, kale, lettuce, mushrooms, mustard greens, okra, onions, parsley, peppers, tomatoes, radishes, snow peas, sauerkraut, spinach, summer squash, swis chard, tomatoes, turnip greens, turnips, scallions
Fruit lowest in carbohydrate
acerola, apricots, avocados, kumquat, lemon, lime, grapefruits, plums, prune
Dairy Products without sugar
butter, cream, cheese, whole milk cottage cheese, cream cheese, milk, ricotta, sour cream, plain whole milk yogurt

Legumes
black-eyed peas, canellini beans, chickpeas, green snap beans, yellow snap beans, kidney beans, lentils, lima beans, peanuts, and soybeans
NUTS & Seeds

The following Vegetarian 30 Day Diet Plan is designed for vegans, those vegetarians who will not eat any animal food whether dairy, fish, seafood, fowl, meat or eggs. If you are a more liberal vegetarian add fish, fowl, seafood, dairy or eggs to the suggested menu you may eat as much as you want of these items since there is usually no carbohydrate in these sources of protein. By now you must hate my repetition, but for some reason I still get frequently asked questions about this. Weird isn't it?

You may substitute any protein with a protein. I have suggested some name brand products that were available on the East Coast and you may have to substitute an item with what products you have available in your area. These name brand products are all vegan. The main idea is to give you a menu suggestion for thirty days and you can freely substitute what you want or have available. You may also substitute a carbohydrate with another carbohydrate as long as you stay with the 30 grams a day limit for thirty days. At the end of the thirty days you may of course, as the diet authority, eat whatever you want. Vegetarians usually have more will power than omnivores but sometimes have difficulty giving up sweets and fruits. Can you do it? It is only for thirty days.

By the way there is a Vegetarian moderator in the Rosacea Diet Users Group who has uploaded a file for vegetarian foods and recipes that is about 80 pages long! She says she is still working on this research paper. You can only access this file and print it if you join the Rosacea Diet Users Support Group. I hope she stays in the group! Her name is

Nadia McLaren and has amazing advice for vegans. I have one post of Nadia's in the chapter, *Frequently Asked Questions*.

30-Day Vegetarian Rosacea Diet Plan

	Vegetarian Menu Eat as much protein as you want! SUBSTITUTE any PROTEIN with a Protein Liberal Vegetarians may add dairy products such as cheese, cream, eggs, or any seafood, fish, or fowl and eat as much as you want!	**Carbohydrate Grams** Just Limit your Carbohydrate To 30 Grams per day!
Day One		
breakfast	at wake up—12 oz. glass of water, Tofu, salt, one cup black coffee or tea, 12 oz glass of water, vitamins	4 inch cube tofu—5.8 grams carbs
Break	12 oz glass of water, celery	2 stalks celery—3.2 grams carbs
Lunch	12 oz glass of water, 1/2 avocado, fresh salad greens, black olives, tomato (vinegar and oil), protein powder, one cup black coffee or tea, 12 oz glass of water	half California avocado—6.5 grams carbs, 4 black olives—1 gram carb, 1 cup of salad greens—2 grams carbs Half tomato—3 grams carbs
Break	12 oz glass of water, celery	2 stalks celery—3.2 grams carbs
Supper	12 oz glass of water, protein powder, asparagus spears, fresh green salad, (vinegar and oil) tea, 12 oz. glass water	4 fresh asparagus spears—2.2 grams carbs 1 cup of salad—2 grams carbs
Day One	Before bed 12 oz glass of water, if you wake up in the night, drink 12 oz glass of water	Total carbohydrate = Less than 30 grams carbs

	Vegetarian Menu Eat as much protein as you want! SUBSTITUTE any PROTEIN with a Pro- tein Liberal Vegetarians may add dairy prod- ucts such as cheese, cream, eggs, or any seafood, fish, or fowl and eat as much as you want!	**Carbohydrate Grams** Just Limit your Carbohy- drate to 30 grams per day!
Day Two		
breakfast	at wake up—12 oz. glass of water, protein powder, one cup black coffee or tea, 12 oz glass of water, vitamins	Zero carbs
Break	12 oz glass of water, cauliflower, mixed nuts	Half cup cauliflower—2.2 grams carbs On and half tablespoons mixed nuts—3.5 grams carbs
Lunch	12 oz glass of water, fresh green salad (vinegar and oil) with tomato, toffutti, one cup black coffee or tea, 12 oz glass of water	Toffutti—2 slices of soy mozzarella slices—2 grams carbs 1 cup of salad greens—2 grams carbs Whole tomato—6 grams carbs
Break	12 oz glass of water, Sunergia Soyfoods, More than Tofu	Sunergia Soyfoods, More than Tofu Indian Masala—2 oz—3 grams carbs
Supper	12 oz glass of water, tofu, cabbage cole slaw or fresh green salad (vinegar and oil) 12 oz glass of water, tea	4 inch cube tofu—5.8 grams carbs, Half cup cole slaw w/dressing —.2.5 grams carbs 1 cup of salad greens —2 grams carbs
Day Two	Before bed 12 oz glass of water, if you wake up in the night, drink 12 oz glass of water	Total carbohydrate = Less than 30 grams carbs

Day Three	Vegetarian Menu Eat as much protein as you want! SUBSTITUTE any PROTEIN with a Protein Liberal Vegetarians may add dairy products such as cheese, cream, eggs, or any seafood, fish, or fowl and eat as much as you want!	Carbohydrate Grams Just Limit your Carbohydrate to 30 grams per day!
breakfast	at wake up—12 oz. glass of water, protein powder, grapefruit, one cup black coffee or tea 12 oz glass of water, vitamins	Half grapefruit—3 in dia.—10.3 grams carbs
break	12 oz glass of water, nuts with celery	1 tablespoon mixed nuts—2 grams carbs 2 stalks celery—3 grams carbs
Lunch	12 oz glass of water, Cole slaw (no sugar in dressing) or fresh green salad (vinegar and oil), Soya Kaas, one cup black coffee or tea 12 oz glass of water	Half cup cole slaw w/dressing—Grams carbs Soya Kaas Mozzarella Style Natural Cheese Alternative—2 oz less than 2 grams carbs 1 cup of salad greens—2 grams carbs
Break	12 oz glass of water, celery, protein powder	2 stalks celery—3 grams carbs
Supper	12 oz glass of water, protein powder, cabbage, fresh green salad (vinegar and oil) 12 oz glass of water, tea	Half cabbage—2.2 grams carbs 1 cup of salad greens—2 grams carbs
Day Three	Before bed 12 oz glass of water, if you wake up in the night, drink 12 oz glass of water	Total carbohydrate = Less than 30 grams carbs

	Vegetarian Menu Eat as much protein as you want! SUBSTITUTE any PROTEIN with a Pro-tein Liberal Vegetarians may add dairy prod-ucts such as cheese, cream, eggs, or any seafood, fish, or fowl and eat as much as you want!	Carbohydrate Grams Just Limit your Carbohy-drate to 30 grams per day!
Day Four		
breakfast	at wake up—12 oz. glass of water, celery and peanut or almond butter, salt, one cup black coffee or tea, 12 oz glass of water, vitamins	2 teaspoons peanut butter or one quarter of ounce almond butter— 6 grams carbs 3 stalks celery— 4.8 grams carbs
Break	12 oz glass of water, fresh cabbage	1 cup raw cabbage— 4.9 grams carbs
Lunch	12 oz glass of water, green salad (vinegar and oil) with green pepper, one cup black coffee or tea 12 oz glass of water	Half cup green pepper— 3 grams carbs 1 cup of salad greens— 2 grams carbs
Break	12 oz glass of water, protein powder	Zero carbs
Supper	12 oz glass of water, cooked cabbage, fresh green salad (vinegar and oil) 12 oz glass of water, tea	1 cup cooked cabbage— 6 grams carbs 1 cup of salad greens— 2 grams carbs
Day Four	Before bed 12 oz glass of water, if you wake up in the night, drink 12 oz glass of water	Total carbohydrate = Less than 30 grams carbs

	Vegetarian Menu Eat as much protein as you want! SUBSTITUTE any PROTEIN with a Pro- tein Liberal Vegetarians may add dairy prod- ucts such as cheese, cream, eggs, or any seafood, fish, or fowl and eat as much as you want!	Carbohydrate Grams Just Limit your Carbohy- drate to 30 grams per day!
Day Five		
breakfast	at wake up—12 oz. glass of water, protein powder, one cup black coffee or tea, 12 oz glass of water, vitamins	Zero carbs
Break	12 oz glass of water, nuts, protein powder	1 tablespoon of Mixed nuts— 2.3 grams carbs
Lunch	12 oz glass of water, fresh green salad (vinegar and oil), tomato, Smart Dogs!, one cup black coffee or tea 12 oz glass of water	1 cup of salad greens—2 grams carbs half tomato—3 grams carbs Smart Dogs! Meat Free soy Protein Links—2 links—10 grams carbs
Break	12 oz glass of water, celery with mixed nuts, protein powder	2 stalks celery—3.2 grams carbs 1 tablespoon mixed nuts—2.3 grams carbs
Supper	12 oz glass of water, salad (vinegar and oil), tomato, protein powder, 12 oz glass of water, tea	salad—2 grams carbs half tomato—3 grams carbs
Day Five	Before bed 12 oz glass of water, if you wake up in the night, drink 12 oz glass of water	Total carbohydrate = around 30 grams carbs

	Vegetarian Menu Eat as much protein as you want! SUBSTITUTE any PROTEIN with a Pro- tein Liberal Vegetarians may add dairy prod- ucts such as cheese, cream, eggs, or any seafood, fish, or fowl and eat as much as you want!	Carbohydrate Grams Just Limit your Carbohy- drate to 30 grams per day!
Day Six		
breakfast	at wake up—12 oz. glass of water, protein powder, one cup black coffee or tea, 12 oz glass of water, vitamins	Zero carbs
Break	12 oz glass of water, celery and nuts	2 tablespoons of Mixed nuts— 4.6 grams carbs 2 stalks celery—3.2 grams carbs
Lunch	12 oz glass of water, cooked spinach, fresh green salad (vinegar and oil) Veggy Singles, one cup black coffee or tea 12 oz glass of water	One cup cooked spinach—6.5 grams carbs 1 cup of salad greens—2 grams carbs Veggy singles (Pepper Jack, cheddar or mazza-rella)—30 grams—1 gram carbs
Break	12 oz glass of water, protein powder and nuts	2 tablespoons of Mixed nuts— 4.6 grams carbs
Supper	12 oz glass of water, fresh green salad (vinegar and oil) with eggplant 12 oz glass of water	Half cup eggplant—4.1 grams carbs 1 cup of salad greens—2 grams carbs
Day Six	Before bed 12 oz glass of water, if you wake up in the night, drink 12 oz glass of water	Total carbohydrate = less than 30 grams carbs

Day Seven	Vegetarian Menu Eat as much protein as you want! SUBSTITUTE any PROTEIN with a Protein Liberal Vegetarians may add dairy products such as cheese, cream, eggs, or any seafood, fish, or fowl and eat as much as you want!	Carbohydrate Grams Just Limit your Carbohydrate to 30 grams per day!
breakfast	at wake up—12 oz. glass of water, protein powder, one cup black coffee or tea, 12 oz glass of water, vitamins	Zero carbs
Break	12 oz glass of water, protein powder	zero carbs
Lunch	12 oz glass of water, peppers, broccoli, fresh green salad (vinegar and oil) with fresh turnip greens, tomato, one cup black coffee or tea 12 oz glass of water	Half cup diced peppers—3 grams carbs Half cup broccoli—3.5 grams carbs Half cup turnip greens—2.6 grams carbs 1 cup of salad greens—2 grams carbs whole tomato—5.8 grams carbs
Break	12 oz glass of water, celery and nuts, protein powder	2 stalks celery—3.2 grams carbs 1 tablespoon mixed nuts—2.9 grams carbs
Supper	12 oz glass of water, asparagus, fresh green salad (vinegar and oil), Smart Deli, 12 oz glass of water	4 asparagus spears—2.2 grams carbs 1 cup of salad greens—2 grams carbs Smart Deli Old World bologna Style Meatless Slices—3 slices—2 grams carbs

Day Seven	Before bed 12 oz glass of water, if you wake up in the night, drink 12 oz glass of water	Total carbohydrate = less than 30 grams carbs

Day Eight	Vegetarian Menu Eat as much protein as you want! SUBSTITUTE any PROTEIN with a Protein Liberal Vegetarians may add dairy products such as cheese, cream, eggs, or any seafood, fish, or fowl and eat as much as you want!	Carbohydrate Grams Just Limit your Carbohydrate to 30 grams per day!
breakfast	at wake up—12 oz. glass of water, Gimme Lean!, scrambled tofu, one cup black coffee or tea 12 oz glass of water, vitamins	Gimme Lean! Meatless Sausage Style—2 oz—4 grams carbs 2 inch cube tofu—2.9 grams carbs
Break	12 oz glass of water, and nuts, protein powder	One and half tablespoons of mixed nuts—3.5 grams carbs
Lunch	12 oz glass of water, fresh green salad (vinegar and oil), protein powder, one cup black coffee or tea 12 oz glass of water	1 cup of salad greens—2 grams carbs
Break	12 oz glass of water, celery with nuts	2 stalks celery—3.2 grams carbs One and half tablespoons of mixed nuts—3.5 grams carbs
Supper	12 oz glass of water, cucumbers, mushrooms, peppers fresh green salad (vinegar and oil), protein powder, 12 oz glass of water	Half cucumber—1.8 grams carbs Half cup mushrooms—2.6 grams carbs Half cup green pepper—3.6 grams carbs 1 cup of salad greens—2 grams carbs
Day Eight	Before bed 12 oz glass of water, if you wake up in the night, drink 12 oz glass of water	Total carbohydrate = around 30 grams carbs

	Vegetarian Menu Eat as much protein as you want! SUBSTITUTE any PROTEIN with a Protein Liberal Vegetarians may add dairy products such as cheese, cream, eggs, or any seafood, fish, or fowl and eat as much as you want!	**Carbohydrate Grams** Just Limit your Carbohydrate to 30 grams per day!
Day Nine		
breakfast	at wake up—12 oz. glass of water, Yves Veggie Cuisine, scrambled tofu, one cup black coffee or tea, 12 oz glass of water, vitamins	Yves Veggie Cuisine the Good Deli Veggie Ham Slices—2 slices— 3 grams carbs 2 inch cube tofu—2.9 grams carbs
Break	12 oz glass of water, nuts, protein powder	One and half tablespoons of mixed nuts—3.5 grams carbs
Lunch	12 oz glass of water, green peppers fresh green salad (vinegar and oil) protein powder, one cup black coffee or tea 12 oz glass of water	One pepper—7.2 grams carbs 1 cup of salad greens—2 grams carbs
Break	12 oz glass of water, protein powder	zero carbs
Supper	12 oz glass of water, salad with whole tomato, (vinegar and oil) 12 oz glass of water, tea	salad—2 grams carbs whole tomato—5.8 grams carbs
Day Nine	Before bed 12 oz glass of water, if you wake up in the night, drink 12 oz glass of water	Total carbohydrate = less than 30 grams carbs

	Vegetarian Menu Eat as much protein as you want! SUBSTITUTE any PROTEIN with a Protein Liberal Vegetarians may add dairy products such as cheese, cream, eggs, or any seafood, fish, or fowl and eat as much as you want!	Carbohydrate Grams Just Limit your Carbohydrate to 30 grams per day!
Day Ten		
breakfast	at wake up—12 oz. glass of water, protein powder, coffee or tea, 12 oz glass of water, vitamins	zero carbs
Break	12 oz glass of water, nuts, protein powder	One and half tablespoons of mixed nuts—3.5 grams carbs
Lunch	12 oz glass of water, tofu, Miso Master Organic Red Miso, fresh green salad (vinegar and oil) one cup black coffee or tea 12 oz glass of water	2 inch cube tofu—2.9 grams carbs Miso Master Organic Red Miso (Traditional soy Paste or Barley Miso)—2 tsp—2 grams carbs 1 cup of salad greens—2 grams carbs
Break	12 oz glass of water, celery and nuts	2 stalks celery—3.2 grams carbs One and half tablespoons of mixed nuts—3.5 grams carbs
Supper	12 oz glass of water, mushrooms, zucchini, spinach fresh green salad (vinegar and oil), protein powder 12 oz glass of water	Half cup mushrooms—1.5 grams carbs Half cup zucchini—2.6 grams carbs 1 cup spinach—6.5 grams carbs
Day Ten	Before bed 12 oz glass of water, if you wake up in the night, drink 12 oz glass of water	Total carbohydrate = less than 30 grams carbs

Day Eleven	Vegetarian Menu Eat as much protein as you want! SUBSTITUTE any PROTEIN with a Protein Liberal Vegetarians may add dairy products such as cheese, cream, eggs, or any seafood, fish, or fowl and eat as much as you want!	Carbohydrate Grams Just Limit your Carbohydrate to 30 grams per day!
breakfast	at wake up—12 oz. glass of water, protein powder, one cup black coffee or tea, 12 oz glass of water, vitamins	Zero carbs
Break	12 oz glass of water, celery with Miso Master Organic Mellow White Soy Paste and nuts	stalks celery—4.8 grams carbs Miso Master Organic Mellow White Soy Paste—2 tsp—3 grams carbs One and half tablespoons of mixed nuts—3.5 grams carbs
Lunch	12 oz glass of water, green beans, fresh green salad (vinegar and oil), one cup black coffee or tea, 12 oz glass of water	Half cup green snap beans—3.4 grams/carb 1 cup of salad greens—2 grams carbs
Break	12 oz glass of water, protein powder	zero carbs
Supper	12 oz glass of water, spinach, fresh green salad (vinegar and oil), Smoke & Fire Soy with Sizzle Herb Smoked Tofu, 12 oz glass of water, tea	One cup cooked spinach—6.5 grams carbs 1 cup of salad greens—2 grams carbs Smoke & Fire Soy with Sizzle Herb Smoked Tofu—half cup—2 grams carbs
Day Eleven	Before bed 12 oz glass of water, if you wake up in the night, drink 12 oz glass of water	Total carbohydrate = less than 30 grams carbs

Day Twelve	**Vegetarian Menu** Eat as much protein as you want! SUBSTITUTE any PROTEIN with a Protein Liberal Vegetarians may add dairy products such as cheese, cream, eggs, or any seafood, fish, or fowl and eat as much as you want!	**Carbohydrate Grams** Just Limit your Carbohydrate to 30 grams per day!
breakfast	at wake up—12 oz. glass of water, Lightlife Fakin Bacon, scrambled tofu, one cup black coffee or tea, 12 oz glass of water, vitamins	Lightlife Fakin Bacon Marinated Smokey Tempeh Strips—3 slices—6 grams carbs 2 inch cube of tofu—2.9 carbs
Break	12 oz glass of water, celery with almond butter	2 stalks celery—3.2 grams carbs Quarter oz almond butter—3.6 grams carbs
Lunch	12 oz glass of water, broccoli, fresh green salad (vinegar and oil), protein powder, one cup black coffee or tea 12 oz glass of water	Half cup broccoli—3.5 grams/carb 1 cup of salad greens—2 grams carbs
Break	12 oz glass of water, celery, protein powder	3 stalks celery—4.8 grams carbs
Supper	12 oz glass of water, asparagus, fresh green salad (vinegar and oil), protein powder 12 oz glass of water, tea	4 asparagus spears—2.2 grams carbs 1 cup of salad greens—2 grams carbs
Day Twelve	Before bed 12 oz glass of water, if you wake up in the night, drink 12 oz glass of water	Total carbohydrate = around 30 grams carbs

Day Thirteen	Vegetarian Menu Eat as much protein as you want! SUBSTITUTE any PROTEIN with a Protein Liberal Vegetarians may add dairy products such as cheese, cream, eggs, or any seafood, fish, or fowl and eat as much as you want!	Carbohydrate Grams Just Limit your Carbohydrate to 30 grams per day!
breakfast	at wake up—12 oz. glass of water, tempeh, one cup black coffee or tea, 12 oz glass of water, vitamins	2 oz. tempeh—7 grams carbs
Break	12 oz glass of water, celery and nuts	2 stalks celery—3.2 grams carbs One and half tablespoons of mixed nuts—3.5 grams carbs
Lunch	12 oz glass of water, eggplant, fresh green salad (vinegar and oil), protein powder, one cup black coffee or tea 12 oz glass of water	Half cup eggplant—4.1 grams/carb 1 cup of salad greens—2 grams carbs
Break	12 oz glass of water, nuts, protein powder	3 oz cheese—1.8 grams carbs One and half tablespoons of mixed nuts—3.5 grams carbs
Supper	12 oz glass of water, mushrooms, fresh green salad, protein powder, (vinegar and oil) 12 oz glass of water, tea	Half cup mushrooms—2.5 gram/carb 1 cup of salad greens—2 grams carbs
Day Thirteen	Before bed 12 oz glass of water, if you wake up in the night, drink 12 oz glass of water	Total carbohydrate = less than 30 grams carbs

Day Fourteen	**Vegetarian Menu** Eat as much protein as you want! SUBSTITUTE any PROTEIN with a Protein Liberal Vegetarians may add dairy products such as cheese, cream, eggs, or any seafood, fish, or fowl and eat as much as you want!	**Carbohydrate Grams** Just Limit your Carbohydrate to 30 grams per day!
breakfast	at wake up—12 oz. glass of water, scrambled tofu with celery and peppers. one cup black coffee or tea, 12 oz glass of water, vitamins	2 inch cube of tofu—2.9 grams carbs 1 stalk celery—1.6 grams carbs Half cup green pepper—3.6 grams carbs
Break	12 oz glass of water, nuts, protein powder	1 tablespoons of mixed nuts—2.3 grams carbs
Lunch	12 oz glass of water, eggplant with fresh green salad (vinegar and oil) one cup black coffee or tea 12 oz glass of water	Half cup eggplant—4.1 grams carbs 1 cup of salad greens—2 grams carbs
Break	12 oz glass of water, celery, South River Certified Organic Sweet Tasting Brown Rice Miso	2 stalks celery—2.4 grams carbs South River Certified Organic Sweet Tasting Brown Rice Miso—1 tsp—2 grams carbs
Supper	12 oz glass of water, Smoke and Fire Soy with Sizzle Lemon Garlic Smoked Tofu and mushrooms fresh green salad (vinegar and oil) 12 oz glass of water, tea	Smoke and Fire Soy with Sizzle Lemon Garlic Smoked Tofu—half cup—3 grams carbs Half cup mushrooms—2.5 gram carbs 1 cup of salad greens—2 grams carbs

Day Fourteen	Before bed 12 oz glass of water, if you wake up in the night, drink 12 oz glass of water	Total carbohydrate = around 30 grams carbs

	Vegetarian Menu Eat as much protein as you want! SUBSTITUTE any PROTEIN with a Pro- tein Liberal Vegetarians may add cheese, cream, eggs, seafood, fish, or fowl as much as you want! Eat as much protein as you want! SUBSTITUTE any PROTEIN with a Pro- tein	Carbohydrate Grams Just Limit your Carbohy- drate to 30 grams per day!
Day Fifteen		
breakfast	at wake up—12 oz. glass of water, scrambled Smoke and Fire Soy with Sizzle Herb Smoked Tofu, one cup black coffee, or tea, 12 oz glass of water, vitamins	Smoke and Fire Soy with Sizzle Herb Smoked Tofu—half cup—2 grams carbs
Break	12 oz glass of water, protein powder, nuts	1 tablespoons of mixed nuts—2.3 grams carbs
Lunch	12 oz glass of water, spinach, fresh green salad with vinegar and oil, one cup black coffee or tea 12 oz glass of water	1 cup spinach—6.5 grams carb 1 cup of salad greens—2 grams carbs
Break	12 oz glass of water, celery with South River Certified Organic Three-Year Barley Miso	3 stalks celery—4.8 grams carbs South River Certified Organic Three-Year Barley Miso—3 tsp—3 grams carbs
Supper	12 oz glass of water, scallions, peppers, and fresh lettuce, grape tomatoes with vinegar and oil 12 oz glass of water, tea	2 tablespoons scallions—2 grams carbs 1 cup of salad greens—2 grams carbs 5 grape tomatoes—3 grams carbs
Day Fifteen	Before bed 12 oz glass of water, if you wake up in the night, drink 12 oz glass of water	Total carbohydrate = less than 30 grams carbs

	Vegetarian Menu Eat as much protein as you want! SUBSTITUTE any PROTEIN with a Protein Liberal Vegetarians may add dairy products such as cheese, cream, eggs, or any seafood, fish, or fowl and eat as much as you want!	Carbohydrate Grams Just Limit your Carbohydrate to 30 grams per day!
Day Sixteen		
breakfast	at wake up—12 oz. glass of water, scrambled Smoke & Fire Soy with Sizzle Lemon Garlic Smoked Tofu, salt, one cup black coffee, or tea, 12 oz glass of water, vitamins	Smoke & Fire Soy with Sizzle Lemon Garlic Smoked Tofu—half cup—3 grams carbs
Break	12 oz glass of water, nuts, protein powder	2 tablespoons of mixed nuts— 4.6 grams carbs
Lunch	12 oz glass of water, kale, protein powder, fresh green salad (vinegar and oil) one cup black coffee or tea 12 oz glass of water	half cup kale—3.4 grams carbs 1 cup of salad greens—2 grams carbs
Break	12 oz glass of water, protein powder	zero carbs
Supper	12 oz glass of water, protein powder, collard greens, fresh green salad with vinegar and oil, one cup black coffee or tea 12 oz glass of water	1 cup collards—9.8 grams carbs 1 cup of salad greens—2 grams carbs 5 grape tomatoes—3 grams carbs
Day Sixteen	Before bed 12 oz glass of water, if you wake up in the night, drink 12 oz glass of water	Total carbohydrate = less than 30 grams carbs

	Vegetarian Menu Eat as much protein as you want! SUBSTITUTE any PROTEIN with a Protein Liberal Vegetarians may add dairy products such as cheese, cream, eggs, or any seafood, fish, or fowl and eat as much as you want!	Carbohydrate Grams Just Limit your Carbohydrate to 30 grams per day!
Day Seventeen		
breakfast	at wake up—12 oz. glass of water, peanut butter with celery, cup black coffee, or tea, 12 oz glass of water, vitamins	2 Tablespoons of peanut butter— 6 grams carbs 2 celery stalks—3.2 grams carbs
Break	12 oz glass of water, nuts, protein powder	2 tablespoons of mixed nuts— 4.6 grams carbs
Lunch	12 oz glass of water, protein powder, green salad (vinegar and oil) with asparagus spears, melted cheddar Veggie Singles, one cup black coffee or tea 12 oz glass of water	4 asparagus spears—2.2 grams carbs 1 cup of salad greens—2 grams carbs Veggie Singles cheddar—30 grams portion—1 gram carbs
Break	12 oz glass of water, celery with peanut butter	2 stalks celery—3.2 grams carbs 2 tablespoons peanut butter— 3.2 grams carbs
Supper	12 oz glass of water, protein powder, raw spinach, fresh green salad (vinegar and oil) 12 oz glass of water, tea	1 cup raw spinach—2.4 grams carbs 1 cup of salad greens—2 grams carbs
Day Seventeen	Before bed 12 oz glass of water, if you wake up in the night, drink 12 oz glass of water	Total carbohydrate = around 30 grams carbs

Day Eighteen	**Vegetarian Menu** Eat as much protein as you want! SUBSTITUTE any PROTEIN with a Protein Liberal Vegetarians may add dairy products such as cheese, cream, eggs, or any seafood, fish, or fowl and eat as much as you want!	**Carbohydrate Grams** Just Limit your Carbohydrate to 30 grams per day!
breakfast	at wake up—12 oz. glass of water, protein powder, salt, one cup black coffee, or tea, 2 oz glass of water, vitamins	Zero carbs
Break	12 oz glass of water, celery	3 celery stalks—4.8 grams carbs
Lunch	12 oz glass of water, turnip, fresh green salad with vinegar and oil, Smart Dogs! and sauerkraut, mustard, one cup black coffee or tea 12 oz glass of water	half cup turnip—.4.3 grams carbs 1 cup of salad greens—2 grams carbs Smart Dogs!—2 links—10 grams carbs
Break	12 oz glass of water, protein powder	zero carbs
Supper	12 oz glass of water, protein powder, spinach, olives, scallions, fresh lettuce salad, vinegar and oil 12 oz glass of water, tea 12 oz glass of water, tea	Half cup spinach—3.25 grams carbs 10 ripe olives—1.2 grams carbs 2 tablespoons scallions—1 gram/carb 1 cup of salad greens—2 grams carbs
Day Eighteen	Before bed 12 oz glass of water, if you wake up in the night, drink 12 oz glass of water	Total carbohydrate = less than 30 grams carbs

Day Nineteen	Vegetarian Menu Eat as much protein as you want! SUBSTITUTE any PROTEIN with a Protein Liberal Vegetarians may add dairy products such as cheese, cream, eggs, or any seafood, fish, or fowl and eat as much as you want!	Carbohydrate Grams Just Limit your Carbohydrate to 30 grams per day!
breakfast	at wake up—12 oz. glass of water, protein powder, one cup black coffee, or tea 12 oz glass of water, vitamins	zero carbs
Break	12 oz glass of water, celery	2 stalks celery—3.2 grams carbs
Lunch	12 oz glass of water, Smoke & Fire Soy with Sizzle BBQ Smoked, cucumbers, tomato, fresh green salad (vinegar and oil) one cup black coffee or tea 12 oz glass of water	Smoke & Fire Soy with Sizzle BBQ Smoked—half cup—3 grams carbs Half cucumber—1.8 grams carbs 1 tomato—5.8 grams carbs, 1 cup of salad greens—2 grams carbs
Break	12 oz glass of water, protein powder	zero carbs
Supper	12 oz glass of water, protein powder, wild rice, mushrooms, fresh green salad (vinegar and oil) 12 oz glass of water	Half cup wild rice—11 grams carbs Half cup mushrooms—1.6 gram carb 1 cup of salad greens—2 grams carbs
Day Nineteen	Before bed 12 oz glass of water, if you wake up in the night, drink 12 oz glass of water	Total carbohydrate = around 30 grams carbs

Day Twenty	**Vegetarian Menu** Eat as much protein as you want! SUBSTITUTE any PROTEIN with a Protein Liberal Vegetarians may add dairy products such as cheese, cream, eggs, or any seafood, fish, or fowl and eat as much as you want!	**Carbohydrate Grams** Just Limit your Carbohydrate to 30 grams per day!
breakfast	at wake up—12 oz. glass of water, protein powder, one cup black coffee or tea, 12 oz glass of water, vitamins	Zero carbs
Break	12 oz glass of water, nuts	2 tablespoons of mixed nuts— 4.6 grams carbs
Lunch	12 oz glass of water, Light Life Foney Baloney, mushrooms with fresh green salad with vinegar and oil, one cup black coffee or tea 12 oz glass of water	Light Life Foney Baloney—3 slices—2 grams carbs Half cup mushrooms—1.6 grams carbs 1 cup of salad greens—2 grams carbs
Break	12 oz glass of water, celery and peanut butter	2 stalks celery—3.2 grams carbs 2 tablespoons cream cheese—6 grams carbs
Supper	12 oz glass of water, Roast beef, broccolio, Brussels sprouts, fresh lettuce, with vinegar and oil 12 oz glass of water, tea	Half cup broccoli—3.5 grams carbs Half cup Brussels sprouts—4.5 gram/carb 1 cup of salad greens—2 grams carbs
Day Twenty	Before bed 12 oz glass of water, if you wake up in the night, drink 12 oz glass of water	Total carbohydrate = less than 30 grams carbs

	Vegetarian Menu	Carbohydrate Grams
Day Twenty One	Eat as much protein as you want! SUBSTITUTE any PROTEIN with a Protein Liberal Vegetarians may add dairy products such as cheese, cream, eggs, or any seafood, fish, or fowl and eat as much as you want!	**Carbohydrate Grams** Just Limit your Carbohydrate to 30 grams per day!
breakfast	at wake up—12 oz. glass of water, scrambled tofu with Light Life Fakin Bacon Marinated Smokey Tempeh, one cup black coffee or tea, 12 oz glass of water, vitamins	2 inch cube tofu—2.9 grams carbs Light Life Fakin Bacon Marinated Smokey Tempeh—3 slices—6 grams carbs
Break	12 oz glass of water, protein powder	Zero carbs
Lunch	12 oz glass of water, Original Tobu Pups, fresh salad greens, black olives, tomato (vinegar and oil) one cup black coffee or tea 12 oz glass of water	Original Tobu Pups—3 links—6 grams carbs 5 black olives—1.2 grams carbs 1 cup of salad greens—2 grams carbs
Break	12 oz glass of water, protein powder	Zero carbs
Supper	12 oz glass of water, asparagus spears with melted Soyco Foods Rice Shreds Cheddar Flavor, fresh green salad (vinegar and oil) 12 oz glass of water, tea	8 asparagus spears—4.4 grams carbs Soyco Foods Rice Shreds Cheddar Flavor—30 gram portion—1 gram carbs 1 cup of salad greens—2 grams carbs
Day Twenty One	Before bed 12 oz glass of water, if you wake up in the night, drink 12 oz glass of water	Total carbohydrate = less than 30 grams carbs

	Vegetarian Menu Eat as much protein as you want! SUBSTITUTE any PROTEIN with a Pro-tein Liberal Vegetarians may add dairy prod-ucts such as cheese, cream, eggs, or any sea food, fish, or fowl and eat as much as you want!	**Carbohydrate Grams** Just Limit your Carbohy-drate to 30 grams per day!
Day Twenty Two		
breakfast	at wake up—12 oz. glass of water, grape-fruit, protein powder, one cup black coffee or tea, 12 oz glass of water, vitamins	Half grapefruit—10.3 grams carbs
Break	12 oz glass of water, protein powder	zero carbohydrate
Lunch	12 oz glass of water, Sunergia Soyfoods More than Tofu Indian Masala, green salad (vinegar and oil) one cup black cof-fee or tea 12 oz glass of water	Sunergia Soyfoods More than Tofu Indian Masala—2 oz.—3 grams carbs 1 cup of salad greens—2 grams carbs
Break	12 oz glass of water, protein powder	zero carbohydrate
Supper	12 oz glass of water, tofu, cabbage, fresh green salad (vinegar and oil) 12 oz glass of water, tea	2 inch cube tofu—2.9 grams carbs 1 cup cabbage—6.2 grams carbs 1 cup of salad greens—2 grams carbs
Day Twenty Two	Before bed 12 oz glass of water, if you wake up in the night, drink 12 oz glass of water	Total carbohydrate = less than 30 grams carbs

	Vegetarian Menu Eat as much protein as you want!	
Day Twenty Three	SUBSTITUTE any PROTEIN with a Protein Liberal Vegetarians may add dairy products such as cheese, cream, eggs, or any seafood, fish, or fowl and eat as much as you want!	**Carbohydrate Grams** Just Limit your Carbohydrate to 30 grams per day!
breakfast	at wake up—12 oz. glass of water, protein powder, one cup black coffee or tea, 12 oz glass of water, vitamins	Zero carbs
Break	12 oz glass of water, nuts	3 tablespoons mixed nuts—7 grams carbs
Lunch	12 oz glass of water, celery and peppers, fresh green salad (vinegar and oil) one cup black coffee or tea 12 oz glass of water	1 stalk of celery—1.6 grams carbs Quarter cup green peppers— 1.8 grams carbs 1 cup of salad greens—2 grams carbs
Break	12 oz glass of water, nuts	3 tablespoons mixed nuts—7 grams carbs
Supper	12 oz glass of water, protein powder, cucumbers, mushrooms, peppers fresh green salad (vinegar and oil) 12 oz glass of water, tea	Half cucumber—1.8 grams carbs Half cup mushrooms—1.6 grams carbs Half pepper—3.2 grams carbs 1 cup of salad greens—2 grams carbs
Day Twenty Three	Before bed 12 oz glass of water, if you wake up in the night, drink 12 oz glass of water,	Total carbohydrate = less than 30 grams carbs

	Vegetarian Menu Eat as much protein as you want!	
Day Twenty Four	SUBSTITUTE any PROTEIN with a Protein Liberal Vegetarians may add dairy products such as cheese, cream, eggs, or any seafood, fish, or fowl and eat as much as you want!	**Carbohydrate Grams** Just Limit your Carbohydrate to 30 grams per day!
breakfast	at wake up—12 oz. glass of water, Gimme Lean!, scrambled tofu, one cup black coffee or tea, 12 oz glass of water, vitamins	Gimme Lean! Meatless Sausage Style—2 oz—4 grams carbs 2 inch cube tofu—2.9 grams carbs
Break	12 oz glass of water, celery	3 stalks celery—4.8 grams carbs
Lunch	12 oz glass of water, Light Life Foney Baloney, fresh green salad (vinegar and oil) one cup black coffee or tea 12 oz glass of water,	Light Life Foney Baloney—3 slices—2 grams carbs 1 cup of salad greens—2 grams carbs
Break	12 oz glass of water, protein powder	Zero carbs
Supper	12 oz glass of water, protein powder, collard greens, cabbage coleslaw, fresh green salad (vinegar and oil) 12 oz glass of water, tea	Half cup collard greens—4.9 grams carbs Half cup cole slaw—4.25 grams carbs 1 cup of salad greens—2 grams carbs
Day Twenty Four	Before bed 12 oz glass of water, if you wake up in the night, drink 12 oz glass of water,	Total carbohydrate = less than 30 grams carbs

	Vegetarian Menu Eat as much protein as you want!	
Day Twenty Five	SUBSTITUTE any PROTEIN with a Protein Liberal Vegetarians may add dairy products such as cheese, cream, eggs, or any seafood, fish, or fowl and eat as much as you want!	**Carbohydrate Grams** Just Limit your Carbohydrate to 30 grams per day!
breakfast	at wake up—12 oz. glass of water, Lightlife Fakin Bacon, scrambled tofu, one cup black coffee or tea, 12 oz glass of water, vitamins	Lightlife Fakin Bacon Marinated Smokey Tempeh Strips—3 slices— 6 grams carbs 2 inch cube of tofu—2.9 carbs
Break	12 oz glass of water, celery	2 stalks celery—3.2 grams carbs 3 tablespoons cream cheese— 1.5 grams carbs
Lunch	12 oz glass of water, Smoke and Fire Soy with Sizzle Herb Smoked Tofu, fresh green salad (vinegar and oil) one cup black coffee or tea 12 oz glass of water,	1 cup of salad greens— 2 grams carbs Smoke and Fire Soy with Sizzle Herb Smoked Tofu— half cup—2 grams carbs
Break	12 oz glass of water, nuts	One and half tablespoons of mixed nuts—3.5 grams carbs
Supper	12 oz glass of water, protein powder, mushrooms and green beans, fresh green salad (vinegar and oil) 12 oz glass of water, tea	Half cup green beans—grams carbs Half cup mushrooms— 1.6 grams carbs 1 cup of salad greens—2 grams carb
Day Twenty Five	Before bed 12 oz glass of water, if you wake up in the night, drink 12 oz glass of water	Total carbohydrate = less than 30 grams carbs

Day Twenty Six	**Vegetarian Menu** Eat as much protein as you want! SUBSTITUTE any PROTEIN with a Protein Liberal Vegetarians may add dairy products such as cheese, cream, eggs, or any seafood, fish, or fowl and eat as much as you want!	**Carbohydrate Grams** Just Limit your Carbohydrate to 30 grams per day!
breakfast	at wake up—12 oz. glass of water, scrambled tofu with celery and peppers, one cup black coffee or tea, 12 oz glass of water, vitamins	2 inch cube of tofu—2.9 grams carbs 1 stalk celery—1.6 grams carbs Half cup green pepper—3.6 grams carbs
Break	12-oz glass of water, protein powder	Zero carbs
Lunch	12 oz glass of water, Smoke and Fire Soy with Sizzle Lemon Garlic Smoked Tofu, fresh green salad (vinegar and oil) one cup black coffee or tea 12 oz glass of water	Smoke and Fire Soy with Sizzle Lemon Garlic Smoked Tofu—half cup—3 grams carbs 1 cup of salad greens—2 grams carbs
Break	12 oz glass of water, celery with Miso Master Organic Red Traditional Soy Paste	2 stalks celery—3.2 grams carbs Miso Master Organic Red Traditional Soy Paste—2 tsp—4 grams carbs
Supper	12 oz glass of water, protein powder, mushrooms, asparagus spears & melted Soyco Foods Rice Shreds Cheddar Flavor, green salad (vinegar and oil) 12 oz glass of water	4 asparagus spears—2.2 grams carbs Half cup mushrooms—1.6 grams carbs Soyco Foods Rice Shreds Cheddar Flavor—30 gram portion—1 grams carb 1 cup of salad greens—2 grams carbs

Day Twenty Six	Before bed 12 oz glass of water, if you wake up in the night, drink 12 oz glass of water	Total carbohydrate = less than 30 grams carbs

Day Twenty Seven	Vegetarian Menu Eat as much protein as you want! SUBSTITUTE any PROTEIN with a Protein Liberal Vegetarians may add dairy products such as cheese, cream, eggs, or any seafood, fish, or fowl and eat as much as you want!	Carbohydrate Grams Just Limit your Carbohydrate to 30 grams per day!
breakfast	at wake up—12 oz. glass of water, scrambled Smoke and Fire Soy with Sizzle Lemon Garlic Smoked Tofu, one cup black coffee or tea, 12 oz glass of water, vitamins	Smoke and Fire Soy with Sizzle Lemon Garlic Smoked Tofu—half cup—3 grams carbs
Break	12 oz glass of water, nuts	One and half tablespoons of mixed nuts—3.5 grams carbs
Lunch	12 oz glass of water, protein powder, Smart Dogs! and sauerkraut, fresh green salad (vinegar and oil) one cup black coffee or tea 12 oz glass of water	Smart Dogs!—2 links—10 grams carbs 1 cup of salad greens—2 grams carbs
Break	12 oz glass of water, celery	3 stalks celery—4.8 grams carbs
Supper	12 oz glass of water, Sunergia Soyfoods More than Tofu Indian Masala, fresh green salad (vinegar and oil) 12 oz glass of water, tea	Sunergia Soyfoods More than Tofu Indian Masala—2 oz.—3 grams carbs Fresh green salad—2 grams carbs
Day Twenty Seven	Before bed 12 oz glass of water, if you wake up in the night, drink 12 oz glass of water	Total carbohydrate = less than 30 grams carbs

	Vegetarian Menu Eat as much protein as you want! SUBSTITUTE any PROTEIN with a Protein Liberal Vegetarians may add dairy products such as cheese, cream, eggs, or any seafood, fish, or fowl and eat as much as you want!	Carbohydrate Grams Just Limit your Carbohydrate to 30 grams per day!
Day Twenty Eight		
breakfast	at wake up—12 oz. glass of water, scrambled tofu, one cup black coffee or tea 12 oz glass of water, vitamins	2 inch cube tofu—2.9 carbs
Break	12 oz glass of water, protein powder	Zero carbs
Lunch	12 oz glass of water, broccoli, fresh green salad (vinegar and oil), Yves Veggie Cuisine the Good Deli Veggie Ham, one cup black coffee or tea, 12 oz glass of water	Yves Veggie Cuisine the Good Deli Veggie Ham—4 slices— 6 grams carbs one cup broccoli—7 grams carbs 1 cup of salad greens—2 grams carbs
Break	12 oz glass of water, celery with nuts	2 stalks celery—3.2 grams carbs One and half tablespoons of mixed nuts—3.5 grams carbs
Supper	12 oz glass of water, protein powder, asparagus with melted Soyco Foods Rice Shreds Cheddar Flavor, fresh green salad (vinegar and oil) 12 oz glass of water, tea	4 spears asparagus—2.2 grams carbs Soyco Foods Rice Shreds Cheddar Flavor— 30 gram portion—1 gram carb 1 cup of salad greens—2 grams carbs
Day Twenty Eight	Before bed 12 oz glass of water, if you wake up in the night, drink 12 oz glass of water	Total carbohydrate = around 30 grams carbs

	Vegetarian Menu Eat as much protein as you want! SUBSTITUTE any PROTEIN with a Protein Liberal Vegetarians may add dairy products such as cheese, cream, eggs, or any seafood, fish, or fowl and eat as much as you want!	**Carbohydrate Grams** Just Limit your Carbohydrate to 30 grams per day!
Day Twenty Nine		
breakfast	at wake up—12 oz. glass of water, scrambled tofu, one cup black coffee or tea, 12 oz glass of water, vitamins	2 inch cube of tofu—2.9 grams carbs
Break	12 oz glass of water, protein powder	zero carbs
Lunch	12 oz glass of water, protein powder, peppers, broccoli, fresh green salad (vinegar and oil), one cup black coffee or tea 12 oz glass of water	Half cup cole slaw—4.25 grams carbs half cup broccoli—3.5 grams carbs Half cup peppers—3.6 grams carbs 1 cup of salad greens—2 grams carbs
Break	12 oz glass of water, celery with nuts	3 stalks celery—4.8 grams carbs One and half tablespoons of mixed nuts—3.5 grams carbs
Supper	12 oz glass of water, protein powder, asparagus, fresh green salad (vinegar and oil) 12 oz glass of water, tea	8 spears asparagus—4.4 grams carbs 1 cup of salad greens—2 grams carbs
Day Twenty Nine	Before bed 12 oz glass of water, if you wake up in the night, drink 12 oz glass of water	Total carbohydrate = less than 30 grams carbs

Day Thirty	Vegetarian Menu Eat as much protein as you want! SUBSTITUTE any PROTEIN with a Protein Liberal Vegetarians may add dairy products such as cheese, cream, eggs, or any seafood, fish, or fowl and eat as much as you want!	Carbohydrate Grams Just Limit your Carbohydrate to 30 grams per day!
breakfast	at wake up—12 oz. glass of water, Gimme Lean! Meatless sausage style and scrambled tofu, one cup black coffee, or tea, 12 oz glass of water, vitamin	Gimme Lean! Meatless sausage style—2 oz—4 grams carbs 2 inch cube tofu—2.9 grams carbs
Break	12 oz glass of water, protein powder	zero carbs
Lunch	12 oz glass of water, Smart Deli Old World Bologna Style Meatless Slices, cucumbers, tomato, mushrooms fresh green salad (vinegar and oil) one cup black coffee or tea 12 oz glass of water	Smart Deli Old World Bologna Style Meatless Slices—3 slices—2 grams carbs Half cup cucumbers—1.8 grams carbs Half cup mushrooms—1.5 grams carbs Half tomato—2.9 grams carbs 1 cup of salad greens—2 grams carbs
Break	12 oz glass of water, celery	2 stalks celery—3.2 grams carbs
Supper	12 oz glass of water, Smoke and Fire Soy with Sizzle BBQ Smoked Tofu, fresh green salad with mushrooms (vinegar and oil), 12 oz glass of water, tea	Smoke and Fire Soy with Sizzle BBQ Smoked Tofu—half cup—3 grams carbs Half cup mushrooms—1.5 grams carbs 1 cup of salad greens—2 grams carbs
Day Thirty	Before bed 12 oz glass of water, if you wake up in the night, drink 12 oz glass of water	Total carbohydrate = less than 30 grams carbs

30 Days to a Lifestyle Diet

If you are convinced that this diet works, you may wish to continue, so I have a few suggestions for the post 30-Day *Rosacea Diet* Plan. If you are not convinced, go ahead and eat all those sugary delights you crave and notice the return of your rosacea and possibly other health problems return. It may take a few days, maybe a week or more but your rosacea will return including any obesity and other health problems. You can control your rosacea with the *Rosacea Diet*. Here are three suggestions for the future:

First, you should be convinced by now that sugar in all its forms is not for you and should be avoided like the plague.

Also, during the 30-Day *Rosacea Diet* Plan I tried to keep your carbohydrate intake to less than 30 grams a day if you followed my suggestions to prove beyond any doubt that rosacea is controlled by a high protein diet and other health problems are reduced or even eliminated. After your thirty-day test, you can now decide how much carbohydrate you can tolerate before your rosacea returns. You can now experiment with any carbohydrate you want, but I suggest you keep your carbohydrate to less than 50 to 100 grams per day for a while. You may be able to tolerate more carbohydrate grams a day but you will just have to experiment to see when your rosacea returns. If you need help on understanding grams and counting them, the best source is *Protein Power* by Michael R. Eades, M.D. and Mary Dan Eades, M.D. *Sugar Busters*! is an excellent source for this as well. And of course Dr. Atkins has many books on the subject too. You may be able to tolerate even more carbohydrate since each individual is a *diet authority* and can decide what is best. Only you can figure out how much carbohydrate you can tolerate and which ones.

Second, if you decide to eliminate sugar in your diet, to control your rosacea or feel healthier, there are many sources of information on how to live without sugar and you can get many books to help at this online source:

http://rosacea-control.com/html/dietbooks.html

I have picked a long list of books that may be interest to you to choose from at the above url. If you still have doubts that a high protein diet is healthy for you, please read *Protein Power* by Drs. Eades or *Dr. Atkin's New Diet Revolution*. These books are available at the above url for your convenience.

Third, what to do about a well balanced diet after the thirty-day test is not as simple as it may seem. You need to achieve a balance in nutrition while at the same time control your rosacea and that is the trick. Experimenting with more carbohydrate like grains and fruits can help you decide what is best for you, so you will have to decide how much you can tolerate through trial and error. Eating a sugary dessert may put you back on the road to your previous diet or eventually after eating sugar for a period of time your rosacea or health problems will return. Taking vitamins as suggested in the chapter on *Vitamins and Supplements* will help bring about in part a well-balanced nutritional diet. You should at least be happy that you have found a way to control your rosacea and feel healthier with the *Rosacea Diet*. You may need additional help from your doctor, other health care professional or nutritionist with their suggestions on diet. Joining the Rosacea Diet Users Support Group at yahoo groups is a great way to discuss the suggestions in these chapters and a way to keep up with the latest information from users of the *Rosacea Diet*. Many have modified eating and drinking with each individual life style and are happy to offer advice. These are a group of *Rosacea Diet authorities*. You may have advice to share. How to join this group is discussed in another chapter. The most important point of the *Rosacea Diet* is that you have learned to control your rosacea and feel healthier with your diet.

You may join by copying and pasting this url into your browser:

http://groups.yahoo.com/group/rosacea-diet-users-support-group

The next chapter gives you a little history of comments I have collected on rosacea over the past four years. The chapter after that gives you more information about the *Rosacea Diet* Users Support Group and then some frequently asked questions. This group is an email support group that has two things in common—we all have this book and we want to talk about it. Hopefully it will motivate you to either join the group discussion or at least be a member and read what others are posting. Why not go to the group site and read the posts since they are public knowledge

History of Posting Rosacea Comments on the Internet

I began posting comments in January 1999 when I began the rosacea-control.com web site. I copied and pasted comments and converted them all to html and posted them for over three and a half years. All the comments from 1999 through January 2002 can be read at my site:

http://www.rosacea-control.com

Upon entering, click on COMMENTS in the left frame or at the top and read the past comments by clicking on the year. There is a lot more information on my site above which categorizes rosacea information into some useful subjects that I post with the latest information on rosacea. The categories include PRODUCTS, RECENT NEWS, PRESCRIPTION, NON-PRESCRIPTION, MEDICAL DOCTORS, IPL, and more.

In November of 1998 David Pascoe of Australia founded his rosacea-support group, http://rosacea.ii.net, which grew into the largest known rosacea support group on planet earth and is another yahoo group and can be seen at this url:

http://groups.yahoo.com/group/rosacea-support/

I would be remiss if I did not mention Pascoe's rosacea-support group. David tries to be non-commercial and claims not to be making any profit on rosacea. We have corresponded over the years through email.

At this printing his group has over 3000 members, which is an amazing feat. David also has his own site on rosacea at this url >

http://rosacea.ii.net/

Since I was involved with my own site posting comments, I ignored Pascoe's group for a long time. There were only a handful of rosacea sites at this period on the Internet. Finally I joined Pascoe's rosacea-support group at yahoo groups in 2001 with the philosophy 'if you can't beat them join them.' After all the number of rosaceans in his group was astonishing. I learned a lot from Pascoe's group and use information gleaned to enhance my own site, rosacea-control.com. I salute what David has done. In August of 2001 I formed the **Rosacea Diet Users Support Group** for users to post comments, improve the diet, and encourage new members and old with any tips or news on rosacea. This group has two things in common, we all have rosacea and we want to control it with our diet. Purchase of the *Rosacea Diet* is required for membership. More on this group is detailed in the next chapter.

In February 2002 I formed the rosaceans group at yahoo groups, which allows anyone to join (as long as they abide by the yahoo group policy) and post comments and I try to mirror the categories on the sister site rosaceans.com. All email comments for rosacea-control.com are now posted at this yahoo group. You should click on POLLS or DATA-BASE in the left frame to see some interesting information. You can join at the following url:

http://groups.yahoo.com/group/rosaceans/

The Rosaceans Group at yahoo allows those rosaceans who do not want to purchase the *Rosacea Diet* a chance to join a group not as large as Pascoe's group. Besides this group is not moderated while Pascoe's is moderated which means the messages are all approved before posted.

There are at the time of the printing of this book 23 yahoo groups on rosacea and you can check the list at this url >
http://groups.yahoo.com/search?query=rosacea&ss=1
Bill Gates has his rosacea groups forming to imitate yahoo >
http://groups.msn.com/
AOL also has rosacea groups if your are a member.

Rosacea Diet Users
Support Group

How to join: go to this url: http://groups.yahoo.com/group/rosacea-diet-users-support-group

In the top right corner, click on 'JOIN THIS GROUP'

Set up a yahoo id and password account that gives you an email account with yahoo. **REMEMBER your yahoo id and password. Write it down.**

You can have all group email go to this yahoo email account you register or you have all group email forwarded to your current email account.

Complete the registration form and click on "Submit This Form."

Note: The Yahoo! ID you choose must be unique. It does not need to match your email address.

To join/subscribe to the *Rosacea Diet* Users Support Group via email:

1. Send a blank email to:

rosacea-diet-users-support-group-subscribe@yahoogroups.com

2. You will receive a subscription confirmation message. Just reply to this message and your subscription will be complete.

Note: The Rosacea Diet Users Support Group is restricted, meaning that the owner or a moderator approves all requests to join. Joining a restricted group sends a message to the owner, who will notify you with an automatically generated email asking you to verify you have the book. You should respond to the owner or a moderator that you have the book. This extra step is required to be approved. Once approved, you will be able to post messages to the group. The exception is if you received an invitation to join, you are pre-approved since your email address is already known and you will not be invited unless someone knows you have the book and invites you.

3. You should receive an email confirming your registration. Be sure to record your Yahoo! ID and password. You will need these to sign into Yahoo! Groups to access group features such as polls and databases, etc.

You may have some questions like these:

What is Yahoo! Groups?

- How much does it cost?

- How do I register?

- How do I start a group?

- How do I transfer my email list to Yahoo! Groups?

- How do I join a group?

- How do I verify my email address?

- How do I unsubscribe from a group?

- Where can I send abuse complaints?

- What is the spam policy in Yahoo! Groups? How do I avoid spam?

- Is it possible for a spammer to gather email addresses from Yahoo! Groups?

- Why am I getting a sign-in error about cookies?

These questions are answered at this url:

http://help.yahoo.com/help/groups/

Setting up your account

Note: You must be signed in with a registered yahoo id and password to use the following features.

- My Preferences allows you to make changes to your account and change your personal preferences. Go here to add email addresses to your account or to verify addresses you've added.
  Some questions you may have are answered at the following url:
  http://help.yahoo.com/help/us/groups/mypreferences/

- The My Groups page is an easy way to manage your groups and subscription settings.
  Some questions you may have are answered at the following url:
  http://help.yahoo.com/help/us/groups/mygroups/

- Click on the Account Info link near the top-right corner to change your Yahoo! account and profile information.

These features are always on the top of the group site

How do I verify my email address?
In order to use an email address for Yahoo! Groups, the address must be verified. The easiest way to set up your account is to use the Mem-

bership Wizard. The wizard will show all of the email addresses you currently have available for use in Yahoo! Groups. Any unverified addresses will be listed at the bottom of the second page. Next to the address will be a "Verify" link. Click on the link to generate a verification email that will be sent to you at that address. Follow the instructions contained in the email to complete the process.

If the email address you wish to use is not listed, click on the Add new email address link.

Common Member Questions

• What are the options for each of my group subscriptions?

• How can I post a message to a group?

• How long does it take for messages to get delivered to the group?

• Why hasn't a message I sent to the group appeared on the web site?

• How can I put message delivery on hold while I'm away and unable to check email?

• Can I post messages from the web site? Can I post from more than one email address?

• Why did I stop receiving email from my group?

• How do I reactivate my Yahoo! Groups account?

The answers to the above questions are found at:
http://help.yahoo.com/help/us/groups/messages

How do I add a new email address to my Yahoo! Groups account?

Answer found at this url:
http://help.yahoo.com/help/us/groups/mypreferences/mypreferences-07.html

How do I unsubscribe from the group?
Answer found at this url:
http://help.yahoo.com/help/us/groups/groups-32.html

What are the options for each of my group subscriptions?
You have these options for your message delivery for each group:

- Individual Emails
  Messages are delivered one at a time to your email inbox. This is the best option if you want to keep up on the latest posts immediately. Email attachments, if included in a message and allowed by your moderator, will be sent directly to you.

- Daily Digest
  Messages are delivered in batches of 25 or daily, whichever comes sooner. This is the best option if you want to receive fewer mail messages and don't need up-to-the minute posts in your inbox. Email attachments are not available in digests.

- Only Special Announcements
  This means you will receive email messages only when the group moderator posts a "Special Announcement" message. This is a good option if you want to pass on day-to-day discussion for very busy groups but do want to receive important updates from the group moderator. Keep in mind that usage by each moderator will vary. (The moderator may choose to never use this feature, in which case you would never receive email messages, or may choose to use it frequently.)

- No Mail/Web Only
  This option puts email message delivery on hold, for example, while you are on vacation. If message archives are available, this option also permits you to read messages at the Yahoo! Groups web site. Note that message archive options are determined by each moderator/owner, and that some groups have no web message archives.

To set any of these options, go to My Groups and choose from the drop-down list of message delivery options for your group.

I suggest you select DIGEST since that is my preference. Try it, you'll like it.

If you have any questions, I will try to answer them if you send an email to the group owner.

Frequently Asked Questions

In previous versions of the *Rosacea Diet* this chapter was extensive to give you an idea of what the Rosacea Diet Users Support Group is all about. Also frequently asked questions were covered here. I have shortened this chapter and tried to cover most of the questions users have raised in all the other chapters of this book. If you really want to read a wealth of information on questions users of the Rosacea Diet have had and the answers that work you need to go to the yahoo group site and click on MESSAGES in the left frame. Then in the SEARCH box at the top of the right frame type in your question or subject and search the archive of messages. If you can't find the SEARCH ARCHIVE box keep, looking in the right frame, it is somewhere. At the printing of this version of the book there were over 2100 posts with all sorts of questions and answers. This archive of posts keeps growing, as does the group. Or if you join the group go ahead and post your own question, but if you don't read what is already posted you will not be up to speed. It is sometimes irritating to the group for a newbie to ask a frequently asked question so why not take some time to research this book first and then the archive before you ask. I don't suggest you have to read all 2100 posts, but you should at least do an archive search for your subject. You should have read this book too since most frequently asked questions are covered somewhere in this book. If you just want to go ahead and read this chapter you will enjoy it and get an idea of what a great support group this really is. There are six moderators who manage the group whenever I am gone and they are all *Rosacea Diet authorities*.

Note: Email addresses have been removed for privacy issues

From: "cschierlmann"
Date: Thu Jan 17, 2002 9:59 am
Subject: Breakfast

I just received the diet and have read over it with much concern. While sweets will be hard to give up, I am more concerned with whole grains, legumes, pasta and fruit. I need some ideas for breakfast instead of meat and eggs. EVERYTHING I normally eat for breakfast is on the banned list and I will go bonkers eating meat and eggs every day. Any suggestions would be appreciated. Thanks—Carol

From: steve
Date: Thu Jan 17, 2002 11:55 am
Subject: Re: [rosacea-diet-users-support-group] Breakfast

Carol:

I can relate to your predicament. I am severely allergic to eggs and can't tolerate cured meats such as bacon so traditional breakfast foods are all out of the question. During the first 30 days of the diet you really MUST give up the grains and fruit to get your skin under control but after that, you may be able to add a few of these back in at breakfast and keep your carbs lower for lunch and dinner. Watch out for whole grain breads because many of them are filled with corn syrup. You really have to read ingredient labels closely. I now look at breakfast foods in a much less traditional manner and I typically go without it. I will sometimes have a piece of chicken later in the morning but earlier than lunch hour. Celery and cream cheese with a few nuts is another breakfast. Perhaps lunch foods interspersed with eggs and cheese, etc. will break up the monotony a little bit.

Best of luck with the diet. Yes, it's hard but I think you'll see good results if you stick to it…and we're here for support! Don't hesitate to ask. steve

From: "Nicola Kamp"
Date: Thu Jan 17, 2002 4:39 pm
Subject: RE: [rosacea-diet-users-support-group] Breakfast

Dear Carol, I suggest you read *Protein Power* to give you some support with your food choice for breakfast. What you are saying is that you are not used to eating such and such foods. So, you have to embrace a different diet and think that you can eat anything for breakfast that is on the list of appropriate foods. You can eat omelets with any kind of vegetable that you may like to eat. Mushrooms, tomatoes, onions, spinach etc. If you are concerned with eating pork or nitrates in breakfast meats, you can always have some sort of roasted meat. I find that eggs are the most appropriate food for breakfast but there is no reason why you couldn't eat fish or poultry. Remember the diet speaks for itself, give it a try and see if your skin is improved. Nicola

From: Nancy Johnson
Date: Thu Jan 17, 2002 5:17 pm
Subject: RE: [rosacea-diet-users-support-group] Breakfast

Trust the diet, give it a try even through the rough spots, and I promise you'll be as grateful on day 28 as I am! I'll NEVER go back to my old eating habits again. I have seen so many beneficial changes in addition to the rosacea control...I feel as if I'm starting out a whole new existence, and I don't get hungry in between meals, even though it seems like I'm not eating much at all. The first week is the toughest...now it's a piece of cake. (OOPS....a piece of string cheese??) Nancy Johnson

From: Debbie Freeberg-Renwick
Date: Thu Jan 17, 2002 8:50 pm
Subject: Re: [rosacea-diet-users-support-group] Breakfast

Boy, I can really relate Carol. It used to be that even if my husband had eggs or meat for breakfast, the smell of them would put my stomach off a bit. I was a toast and jam or cream of wheat and black tea with cream and sugar kind of gal. When I read your email I realized that I don't even think twice about it anymore. I have chicken and some vegetables for breakfast with no queezy feeling whatsoever. I look forward to it. In fact my stomach rarely feel queezy at all and it used to a lot. I just realized that. But at first when I was doing this diet, I remember it was really hard. I cheated and had decaf black tea with cream and stevia. It gave me some familiar reference point and some sweetness. I have gotten a sense from what I have read of other's experiences, that I was/is more addicted to sweet tastes and carbs in general than most. I used to eat frequent small meals high in carbs or else black tea or diet soda to keep going. From the outside people thought my diet to be very moderate and healthy, but that was not how it felt. I constantly had a feeling I was running on empty. Now, when I stick to the diet, my energy is even and although I still have frequent small meals, they are high protein. And I often find my energy can outlast that of my high carb friends. I have come to think of eating as refueling instead of jump starting—a crude analogy, but hopefully you get my drift. So, I know some of this is a bit off your topic question, but I thought maybe someone else's experience might help in some way. Best of luck and stay in touch. Debbie

---

From: Nancy Johnson
Date: Thu Jan 17, 2002 9:44 pm
Subject: Re: [rosacea-diet-users-support-group] Breakfast

"Debbie Freeberg-Renwick"

I have come to think of eating as refueling instead of jump starting I really like your "refueling" analogy...that's exactly what it's like. I never feel hungry like I used to when I was ready to stuff something in my mouth the minute I got home. Now I look forward to eating but can wait if necessary, and my energy is very even and controlled instead of up and down. I'm more of a nibbler than a "gulper" now...Nancy Johnson

---

From: monica page
Date: Fri Jan 18, 2002 10:04 am
Subject: Re: [rosacea-diet-users-support-group] Breakfast

My breakfast (and usually lunch and dinner) are broccoli and tofu w/tamari or something like that. My diet is radically different from my spouse and all my friends, but what's the alternative? Advanced Rosacea, broken blood vessels, etc. Those thoughts keep me in line. Besides, I too have eaten enough carbs and sugar until now to last me a lifetime.

The benefits of my "weird" diet are tremendous, however. I look 10 years younger, my energy and emotions are more pleasant and consistent.

Wishing you the best, it's not easy. We're very lucky to have this group. Thanks to everyone. Monica

lori ashbaugh wrote >

---

the diet did not help my rosacea, though i lost weight though, which was nice and feel like i have a little more energy my rosacea and flaring remains the same

thanks, anyway

From: Debbie Freeberg-Renwick
Date: Fri Jan 18, 2002 9:32 pm
Subject: Does/can the diet work?

Hi Lori,

The internet is weird here today so I will write a bit and send it and then write again. I just lost a long letter. I hate it when that happens...If I was you, and of course I am not, but if I was, I would try to give it a little longer. It took me a LONG time to see really good results that lasted. I can't even remember how long. I attribute this to two things. One, my addiction to carbs. I found that this really colored my perspective on everything. I felt it was unfair that I had to do this weird diet to have good looking skin when everyone around me could pig out and look great. I totally was not taking responsibility. Sounds like a very adolescent attitude I know. Embarrassing thing is that I am 48 and have 2+masters degrees. Addictions I have come to realize are very insidious, sneaky beasts that block our vision and I feel I am still wrestling with it. I feel much akin to alcoholics, and I didn't even drink before. I am going to send this now and start continue in another email...

From: Debbie Freeberg-Renwick
Date: Fri Jan 18, 2002 9:54 pm
Subject: Does/can the diet work? #2

continuing...So this 'need' for carbs created some blind spots for me. It was not a real conscious thing at all. It took time for me to uncover this tendency in myself. So that is one reason it took me a long time to see results. Another reason is that it is just a fact that MANY things have some form of sugar in them. It took me a year or so before I realized that my salt had sugar in it. I had never thought to look. All iodized salt has dextrose in it. Dextrose holds the iodine in the salt particles. I have said for a long time I was going to check out everything before it went into my mouth, but things STILL sneak past my better judgement, and I pay every time. Sometimes I feel like a real idiot. Like lately when I had a 15+hour flight to do. I packed all my meals and snacks in a nice insulated bag. I never eat anything that the airlines offers but water and soda water (and then I ask to see the can). I took my usual meals and snacks of walnuts and a recently rediscovered food—dulce. It is salty and sort of reminiscent of potato chips and has lots of minerals and vitamins. Somehow I NEVER thought to look up the carbs on it. To make a long story short, it is 45% carbs and because it is very condensed, a big handful can be 30 carbs. So, for 3 days I ate my dulce snack AND my 30 carbs of broccoli and lettuce. Four days later my skin was a MESS. Plus my skin was riding the edge anyway—I had knowingly eaten too much of the veggies I usually eat over Christmas, trying to pacify something that was freaking out watching everyone around me eat all my favorite carbs. I am in humble awe at my ability to space out on these things...Another thing is, I can't eat all the stuff Brady suggests starting out with. It is so individual, I don't think anyone could come up with a diet that would 100% work for everyone. But it is a good starting point. I have found I can't eat dairy, spicy things, fried things, pork, and seafood. It is a drag, but my skin looks clear and as I think it was Nancy who said it, I look much younger. Most think I am at most 35. That is cool. So my point is? Try to look carefully at what you have eaten and what you are eating. Maybe this diet isn't for you. But maybe it is, and maybe it will take more 'tweaking' to get it to a workable place. Just the fact that you feel better in other ways could be a sign. Could be that it is working from the inside out, to put it in very unscientific words. The best of luck to you. Sincerely, Debbie

From: steve
Date: Sat Jan 19, 2002 10:10 am
Subject: Re: [rosacea-diet-users-support-group] Re: Lori

Lori:

A couple of things to add to what Debbie had to say.

I found that the diet took more than 30 days to see definitive results. I thought it MIGHT be a little better after the first 30 days but I wasn't convinced. But I stayed on it because I was losing weight (a good thing for me). It took another 30 days before I really felt the diet was having a positive effect on my skin. Even after that, I have had breakouts—even severe ones—as I tweaked the diet to exclude other foods that I cannot tolerate. We've seen a wide variety of other unique individual trigger foods through this group. I have been on the diet for about 13 months and I feel I'm still refining my diet.

Another problem I have—and I know at least a few others have as well—is stress. I have a job that can at times be very stressful. During these times, even keeping my carbs below 20 grams a day will not control my rosacea. There was also a two-month period of time when I was buying a new house that I tried to be conscious of keeping my stress level in check that I could not control my rosacea with the diet. Two or three days after I closed on the house, my rosacea was gone. I've even considered leaving my job for a simpler, less stressful way of life. That may seem silly to prevent a pink face but rosacea affects so much more than my physical appearance; it affects my self image and general sense of well being.

I would encourage you to stay with the diet for awhile, experiment a bit and keep looking for other things that might be affecting your rosacea. I think you'll eventually find a balance that works for you. Hang in there!

steve

From: Nancy Johnson
Date: Fri Jan 18, 2002 7:08 pm
Subject: Re: [rosacea-diet-users-support-group] Breakfast

Lori, Brady, and everyone...

This is day 29 for me, and I can honestly say that this diet is the best thing I've done for myself in all my 55 years. Here are the changes I've seen in this brief time:

Joint pain, which previously had me in physical therapy and in repeated doctor visits, is gone. Completely gone. I now have full range of motion in my neck (an MRI had shown arthritis). My knees don't make that cellophane crackle when I walk up the stairs, and I don't say "Oh, my back" every time I try to straighten up. I don't know how much of that can be attributed to the diet itself and how much to the water consumption (I'm sure I was chronically dehydrated before the diet), but whatever it is, it has been a blessing beyond words. A stubborn toenail fungus has cleared up. The doctor had said that it would take a year at least with oral medication, and even then might not go away. It's gone. I think I was feeding it with the sugar. My skin has a finer texture than it has had in YEARS. I also changed most of the topicals that I was using, and the emu oil has made a big difference, but again I think the water has been the biggest factor, and without this diet I would NEVER have given up my Dr. Pepper for WATER. I've lost over ten pounds...not one of my goals, but I look and feel better and more energetic and more "centered" than I can remember ever feeling before. I really notice it at school...I teach middle school kids, and even THEY can't ruffle my new serenity! I don't crave sugar any more, and I don't think there was a person on earth who was a bigger sugar fiend than I was. When we ate out, I would order desert first and eat it while I waited for the dinner. I could polish off half a cherry pie in one evening. I didn't have a weight problem, but now that I've lost some weight, I can see how much better I look with skin over muscle instead of over fat. My husband is beginning to eat healthier now that he's fixing my meals for me most of the time. He's seen the big difference in my overall condition, so I haven't had to say a word to convince him. I've discovered tea! I never tried tea or coffee in my life, but finally tried tea as a bit of change from all the water, and it has been a delightful new addition to my day. (Check out www.strandtea.com) My favorite so far is rooibos, filled with vitamins, nutrients, and antioxidants. I have a very consistent energy level...not the ups and downs of hunger and "too-fullness" that I used to have. I don't get "hungry" and I have broken the "I'm sitting down therefore I should be eating" habit. I'm looking forward to the next 30 days to see if a continuation of the diet (with a slight increase in carbs) will bring even more benefits. I have an appointment with my doctor on February 18, and she doesn't know that I've been doing this. I can't wait to see what she says. I'm going to offer to loan her Dr. Nase's book. If she doesn't seem interested in learning more about rosacea, then I may just start looking around for another doctor. The diet DOES work. I still can't control the hot room problem at school...and in other places...but I will control the things I can and try not to worry about the things I can't control. Thanks again, Brady...I don't remember how I happened to stumble onto the rosacea list in the first place, but it has led me to a new and wonderful point in my life! Nancy Johnson

---

To: Rosacea Diet Users Support Group
From: Lee Everett
Date: Tue Oct 2, 2001 3:54 pm
Subject: Comments

Hello to all members...

I'm on my soapbox today to say that I am feeling very dismayed by all the emails I've read......the subjects being creams, medicine, lotions, antibiotics etc.

Why does everyone feel so compelled to use all these items? The Rosacea Diet has given us 'keys to the kingdom of healthy skin". I have had Rosacea for two years prior to finding the Rosacea Diet and I also have discoid Lupus eruptions on my face and believe me I have not been a 'happy camper' about having both conditions to resolve. I couldn't even tolerate having sunlight in my house or the glare from my computer....even while I used medicinal creams and gobs of sunblock. It was at the height of my frustration that I began to research the web and found this diet......AND IT WORKS LIKE A CHARM!

It's been two months now and my rosacea barely is visible and the deep red raw Lupus eruptions are beginning to fade. All my window shades are pulled up and no more sunblock. I still wear a sunhat when I go out, minimal sunblock and the greatest thing of all is that my face doesn't feel like its on fire.

Here are a few things I have learned.....antibiotics wreck havoc with the intestinal flora and eventually the entire digestive tract......sugar intensifies this imbalance and so does yeast of any kind and also aged cheeses and vinegar.....information on this can be researched on the web and is often classified as candida. If you read *Sugar Blues* you'll learn how insidious sugar is.

After trying the rosacea diet and feeling awesome at the results.....I learned (for myself) high protein, minimal to no sugar every day, two slices of bread a week, no aged foods or vinegar helps in great measure. I reflected on a job I had many years ago in a convalescent hospital.... patients were give Ensure.... a high protein liquid...to heal open wounds.... and it seemed like magic to watch the open wounds heal...so, in that reflection plus the info Brady shared with us, I concluded (for myself) that proteins have a far greater benefit then I ever realized.

I really hope that my words have touched someone enough to re-evaluate their daily selection of foods....

Lee Everett

From: "denimaddict"
Subject: diet and rosacea

Hello! I have been sitting back reading all of your e-mails and waiting for the right time to participate. You see, I have been on the rosacea diet for almost three weeks and my face is almost entirely clear and my redness is 95% gone. This diet is not easy, but I followed it to the letter. I often read many of your notes claiming to be on the diet but off of it a meal a day...You are not on the diet!! I see people asking if they can eat this or that food item...it's pretty clear in the diet what you can and can't eat.

Don't make it so complicated. I thought that this group was for the people on the diet and his other group just for those with rosacea, but I find alot of talk that doesn't seem as though the diet has been examined. Anyway, this may or may not have worked faster for me than for some of you, but I made a pact with myself to give it the thirty days and it has really paid off! I have to say it is difficult managing the cravings for so many things not allowed on the diet, but looking in the mirror and seeing the results really makes it all worthwhile.

I went to my dermatologist this week and he stood there with his mouth open, and for the first time, speechless! I do hope that those of you who have not really given this diet your full and honest attempt, will think again.

Well I hope I haven't offended anyone...it's just that I want you guys to have the same success that I have found. Thank you Brady!

Marianne

From: Brady

Marianne,

thanks for the post. your experience is what I have always found out myself. when I go off my own diet I have a rosacea flare. it is difficult when friends and family offer those tempting delights. I am a sucker for tortilla chips, particularly red hot blues. I pay for it every time on my my face! I am the first to recognize my own diet is extremely difficult, but my face is worth the sacrifice and setting an example is an obvious reason to stay on my own diet!

you are right, the rosaceans group at yahoo which right now has been more active than ever is for rosaceans who want to talk about anything but controlling their rosacea with diet. right now, this group is in a big discussion on diet triggers!

the RDUSG has two things in common. we all have rosacea and we are trying to control it with diet. however, I have no objection to the discussions changing to IPL, drugs, non-prescription treatments and the like. we need to keep up with what may help any of us.

Brady

From: Brady Barrows
Date: Fri Jun 6, 2003 11:14 am
Subject: diet and rosacea
---In rosacea-knowledge@yahoogroups.com, skwpt <skwpt@y...> wrote:
> > 05 Jun 2003 wrote (with heavy snipping on skwpt's part):

> There are quite a few rosaceans on another board (roeacea
> diet support) who are eating low carb and are seeing
> vast improvements in their symptoms. I am one of them,
> but I eat closer to 100 grams of cabrohydrate a day
> than the recommended 30.

Just some clarification on the recommended 30 carbohydrate a day you mention above. This recommended restriction on carbohydrate per day for thirty days is to prove beyond any doubt that this diet controls rosacea, which it has for hundreds of users. After the thirty days the recommendation is for each rosacean to determine how many carbohydrate to eat, as much as desired, hence the need for a rosacea-diet-users-support-group. Each member has modified the rosacea-diet to his/her own particular rosacea condition, eating and drinking food/drink individually, which is a great support group since we all have this in common and can give tips to each other.

> It frustrates me that so many medical professionals
> believe that diet has no (or little affect) on Rosacea...

There are a growing number of physicians who do believe diet is a factor in rosacea though admittedly few. Nicholas V Perricone, M.D. and Christiana Northup, MD are two you mention among others.

This should encourage those who desire to use diet to control rosacea. The debate over 'elimination diets' is hot, yet my contention is that this diet is a life style change, not an elimination diet. Since there is such an ongoing debate among physicians about diet and health, the aftershocks of this spills over into groups like rosacea-support and rosacea-knowledge. Rosaceans in general do not want to change their life style diet and site physicians who browbeat Dr. Perricone, Dr. Atkins, Drs Eades, Dr. Northup, and others who discuss diet and health. But guess what rosaceans in every yahoo group eventually bring up over and over again? Diet. Yet the debate over it is endless simply because rosaceans want to eat and drink what they want to eat and drink. It is a 'have your cake and eat it too' mentality. We all suffer from this mentality but a few rosaceans realize that you don't have to either have the cake or eat it and your rosacea improves.

Brady Barrows

From: Pam Tobey
Subject: [rosacea-diet-users-support-group] Re: diet and rosacea I'd say this really hits the nail on the head! The attackers always say that diet can't change rosacea or skin, when we know it does! LOL. And they always bring up the myths about lo carb diets as if they were truth and say there are no studies. I have an old Atkins brochure which lists 5 medical studies, funded by groups as different as the Atkins Center, the government and the Am.

Heart Assn! And there have to be many more, as well as a few ongoing ones I've heard about.

My problem is the crux of brady's comment, that it is up to the rosacean and the will power to change. I "fell off the wagon" recently and the rosacea flares got back to their old "badness." I've climbed back on the wagon and started over and just have to try and hang on when that wagon hits a bump in the road! LOL. I haven't had as hard a time with the carbs, as in bread and that kind, but it's the sugars, like aspartame and wine that are really hard to give up, for me.

Pam in D.C.

From: Suzanna Edgar

Subject: RE: [rosacea-diet-users-support-group] Re: diet and rosacea I totally agree with both these messages—it is horrifying that doctors do not understand or wish to understand the link between skin and diet. We all know that it is because of money—the doctors have to push the antibiotics/topicals to satisfy the drug companies. This is the reason why it has become so important for me to go back to school and get a degree in nutrition/naturopathy (I work in the investment industry!) I really want others to know a safer and effective way to clear the skin and obtain a much healthier lifestyle at the same time. This diet has been the only thing that has worked for me—it is key for me to keep my carb levels to just below 30 grams a day—any higher and I break out and flush.

So thanks to Brady for this miraculous discovery. As I have mentioned many times before—I like to combine this super low carb diet with food choices from the blood type diet. The two of them work wonders for my skin. I have to be very careful not to go over the carb limit. After a while, one gets used to this diet and it gets much easier.

Suz

From: Jyoti

Hi, Brady,

I think I am already signed up with Yahoo, and thought I was already also part of your group. Dunno how I got so confused. I already have purchased the Rosacean Diet book, and am trying to adhere to it, but it is (as he warns us) VERY VERY hard to follow. But I should be grateful that my rosacea is not so noticeable right now, and there is no pain at all.† It is hard to always remember to wear my hat outside in our very hot summer (Texas) but I do try. What helps me is to adhere religiously to my chosen 'treatment' option, and to also try hard to adhere to the diet. I have to say that it was a very big surprise to me when I realized what I had! I've not had skin problems before now.

(I'm 63) I always had very good, almost translucent skin, and was (I'm afraid) very vain about it. Well, I'm not vain anymore, so maybe that's a good thing!

Warmly—Jyoti

From: Suzanna Edgar
Subject: RE: [rosacea-diet-users-support-group] FWD: Welcome Welcome Jyoti,
I also found the diet quite an adjustment at the beginning. I have been 100% compliant now for about 2 months—I sort of half started a while ago, but am now very strict with it. It has become quite a natural way of eating to me now—so don't worry you will adjust. My body has become very used to not having sugar. My skin is totally clear now after months of awful redness, pimples and discomfort. It actually only took 2 weeks for my skin to clear. I have had several people comment on how beautiful my skin is and they asked me what products I use!! I told them that I do it all through diet—which to be honest is true. They cannot believe that I actually have a skin condition! I do avoid harsh skin products as I know my rosacea skin is very sensitive—but the glow really comes from the diet! The key is to keep the carbs to less than 30 grams a day—and then after 30 days, see how much your skin can tolerate. My skin really doesn't like any more than 30. I eat lots of fresh veggies and just a little fruit and lots of fish, eggs and meat. I have far more energy than I had before and sleep very well now—so there are all sorts of benefits to this diet.

So—welcome and just know that you are on your way to super clear skin again!

Suz.

From: Nadia
Subject: Re: att. Suzanne Edgar/How is it possible?
Suz wrote:…how it is possible to eat LOTS of veggies and at the same time keep your carb intake below 30 grams a day?

It's not easy to keep below 30g, especially so for vegetarians. And if you are vegan it starts to get plain tedious. Creativity is required.

A serious penalty with the 30-day diet is that you will probably not get enough protein—low carbs and high protein just don't come in the same vegetarian food, except for tofu. But you will survive the month even if you are a vegan (and cannot eat eggs or hard cheese).

Also see Lowcarb Vegetarian Protein Sources http://www.immuneweb.org/lowcarb/food/protein.html for good material on food balancing).

The firmer the tofu, the more protein and the fewer carbs. Use the firmest "cotton" tofu if you can find it. It's the type usually available packed in rectangular tubs and immersed in water, in refrigerator cases in Chinese stores and produce departments of regular supermarkets. Ask for GM-free. Firm tofu is dense and solid and holds well in stir-fry dishes, soups, or on the grill. Soft tofu is an excellent choice for recipes that call for blended tofu. Silken tofu is made by a slightly different process that results in a creamy, custard-like product. Silken tofu works well in pureed or blended dishes. Different from milk-based products, "light" tofu products have fewer carbs.

There are now also tofu-based substitutes for yogurts, cheeses, spreads, milks, creams and icecreams. Count carbs from the label.

NB: tempeh is also made from soya beans but has 17 g carbs per 100g as compared with 1–5g for tofu. Wait until your 30 days are up, but perhaps try textured vegetable proteins (TVP) made from soya and quorn (mushroom protein). Seitan is often called the "meat substitute". It is made from wheat gluten and like quorn and TVP contains around 8g carbohydrate per 100g.

Remember the 30g carbs per day limit is only for 30 days so that you can verify the response of your rosacea to the diet. Then you can increase carbs. In my view, vegetarians can increase quite a lot because at least one third of carbs in vegetables is fibre, ie non-digestible and non-sugar forming. Look here for Carbohydrate in a Vegetarian Diet http://www.vegetarian-diet.info/vegetarian-diet-carbohydrate.htm

See the list below with the carb content of vegetables and fruits.

Here's some ways to make a limited food range more interesting

Try different cooking methods for vegetables: stir-fry, braised, roasted, sauted in brown butter, microwaved with cheese or cream topping (+/-lemon and chives), raw with dips and dressings, sauted and blended with cream for soups (hot and cold)

Practice cooking tofu in different ways. Add taste with frying, aromatic oils, garlic and herb butters a little seasoning, miso, dressing, herbs, spices (not hot) soy sauce, salsas (not hot), pestos and other suitable accompaniments

Help fill yourself with liquid, eg saute and cook the veggies in water and blend to make soup. Chilled soups are good in summer.

If you are cooking for family or guests, look here for recipes with carbohydrate counted (you can adjust quantity interactively) http://www.recipezaar.com/browse/index.zsp?pg=1&path=0FC15C11F06B These meals are low in carbohydrate; add high carb extras, like sweetcorn and fruits, for the others at the table.

Good eating

Nadia

From: "Connie Rice"
I got so much out of the group, Brady, I cannot begin to tell you how much you changed my life. Regardless of rosacea, I needed to change my diet drastically for overall good health and that's what I've done. I feel like I've finally found a balance between food and skin care that keeps my rosacea totally manageable without prescriptions, and that is all thanks to you. Please never underestimate the amazing transformational affect you have had on many peoples' lives.

Take care,

Connie

Polls and Databases on Rosacea

In the Rosacea Diet Users Support Group and in the Rosaceans Group there are polls and database features members enjoy. In this chapter I have the results of the polls and databases in August 2003 at both yahoo group sites. These results are not scientific and are subject to change if new members participate in these features and vote or add records. Yet as you read the results in this chapter you will do doubt find the results interesting and may help you find information on controlling your rosacea. Many of the products used to control rosacea are found on my website.[1] Click on PRESCRIPTION, NON-PRE-SCRIPTION, IPL or other page to find more information. Links to these products can be found if you search there.

You may learn more about how to use polls or database features at these urls >
Polls
http://help.yahoo.com/help/us/groups/polls
Database
http://help.yahoo.com/help/us/groups/database

These are some of the poll questions and the results. While the polls or databases are not scientific results, they are certainly interesting.

Besides the *Rosacea Diet*, What other treatment(s) do you use?
26% Use prescription medication
16% Linda Sy Skin Care Products

---

1.   http://www.rosacea-diet.com

208

18% Flaxseed Oil²
12% Grapeseed Extract
4% IPL
4% Rosacea LTD-III
2% Sher System
2% Andrzej Wedrychowski's Formula

Have you found that sugar substitutes trigger your rosacea?
8.33 %—YES
25 %—NO
8.33 %—Some sugar substitutes
50 %—I avoid sugar substitutes
8.33 %—I don't know
DATABASE
What other treatment not listed in the Polls do you use to treat your rosacea?
Typical record >
I take a Minocycline every day I wash my face with Plexion twice a day and I use Noritate cream every morning

Other Databases available >
Recipes
Sugar Free Products
Vegetarian Products or Suggestions
Recipes—Vegetarians
What sugar substitute triggers your rosacea?

Files
Vegan and vegetarian notes
An updated list of the sugar and sugar substitutes to avoid during the 30 day Rosacea Diet Plan
GT's Rosacea Diet Humor

---

2.   not a topical but an oil to ingest

Rosaceans Group at Yahoo groups

Polls
Most popular poll >
How do you treat your rosacea?
Prescription Medications—29%
Non-Prescription Medications—Topicals or pills—17%
Non-prescription soap—14%
Vitamins—12%
Diet—9%
Cosmetics—6%
IPL—5%
Herbal treatments 4%
Laser—3%
Accupuncture 1%

What kind of treatment do your use to control your rosacea?
Traditional physician treatments—40%
Alternative non-physician treatments—23%
Both of the above treatments—37%

What non-prescription treatments do you use to control your rosacea?
Flaxseed Oil—14%
Rosacea Diet © 9%
Linda Sy's Skincare Products—9%
Jojoba Oil—8%
Grapeseed extract—8%
Eucerin—8%
Rosacea LTD-III—7%
Rosaceacare Skincare Products—7%
Purple Emu—6%

Rosacea Resolved Cream—4%
Sulphur soap—3%
Dermalogica—3%
Sher System Products—2%
Rosaceacure—2%
Florasone—2%
ELICINA® CREAM—1%
Andrzej Wedrychowski's Formula—1%
Acne-Rosacea.co.uk Products—1%
Abby's Herb Company—1%
Natures's Gift Rosacea Synergy—1%

Second & Third poll,
Cetaphil 11 votes
Paula's Choice—3 votes
VitaKsolution—2 votes
ZenMed—2 votes
Cutanix—2 votes
Emu Oil—2 votes
Dermal K—1 vote
Colloidal Silver 1 vote
Ombrelle—1 vote
Rosacea Cream—1 vote
RosaceaGon—1 vote
SkinFix ®—1 vote
SpectroJelÆ—1 vote
Vanicream—1 vote
Vitamin B3—1 vote
Pevonia RS2 for Rosacea—1 vote

How many rosacea treatments (prescription or non-prescription) do you use?
One—24%
Two—36%
Three—21%
Four—13%
More than five—6%

Most Voted Prescription Medications >
Metrogel, Metrocream, MetroLotion, (metronidazole), Noritate, Doxycycline hyclate,TETRACYCLINE

Do you suffer from depression due to rosacea?
Yes—53%
No—20%
Maybe—27%

Database tables to view on the rosaceans group site >
Physician Database
Famous Rosaceans
What treatment for rosacea did NOT work for you?

Physician Treatment

As my legal disclaimer states at the beginning of this book, you may need additional treatment for your rosacea from a physician or health care practitioner to control your rosacea. First and foremost a physician should diagnose you with rosacea. One problem that has come up with rosaceans is that rosacea may be misdiagnosed for other diseases. More information on this can be found at this url >

http://www.rosaceans.com/html/tip.html#mis

It is possible also to have other skin diseases along with rosacea,[1] so seeing a physician is important not only to diagnose rosacea but also to check for other conditions. There is a list of physician search engines at this url >

http://www.rosaceans.com/html/md.html

A must have guide on rosacea is Dr. Nase's book[2] when being treated by a physician which offers the most comprehensive information in book form to date. A review of his book can be found at this url >

---

1. For an example, "While the rosacea and seborrheic dermatitis are different skin disorders, sometimes they can coexist at the same time. Approximately 35% of people with rosacea have seborrheic dermatitis which makes for an even more sensitive skin condition." Source >
    http://internationalrosaceafoundation.org/dermatitis_factor.html

2. "See your doctor. It's easy to mistake skin disorders and doctors know best how to identify and treat rosacea."—*Rosacea—What You should Know,* page 8, Galderma Laboratories, Inc.

http://www.rosaceans.com/html/nase.html

There are so many physician treatments for rosacea. A partial list includes prescription medication[3], IPL[4], Laser[5], ETS[6], nitric oxide inhibitors[7], Pycnogenol[8], WobenzymeN™[9], Botox™[10], and other treatments.[11] This book is not intended to comment on these treatments. These are mentioned to simply inform you. I have included links to information available for you and recommend Dr. Nase's book if you use physicians to treat your rosacea. Dr. Nase comments on most, if not all of these treatments for rosacea and a whole lot more. The National Rosacea Society[12] in the USA and the Rosacea Awareness Program[13] in Canada both offer physician treatment information for rosacea which is the only information offered by both these organizations.

3.   For a list of links on prescription medication for rosacea check this url >
     http://www.rosaceans.com/html/pre.html—See also >
     http://internationalrosaceafoundation.org/prescription.html
4.   http://www.rosaceans.com/html/ipl.html—Also see *Beating Rosacea Vascular, Ocular & Acne Forms, A Must-Have Guide to Understanding & Treating Rosacea*, Geoffrey Nase, Ph.D., Nase Publications, 2001, pages 178–186
5.   *Beating Rosacea Vascular, Ocular & Acne Forms, A Must-Have Guide to Understanding & Treating Rosacea*, Geoffrey Nase, Ph.D., Nase Publications, 2001, pages 173–178, 186–7
6.   Endoscopic Transthoracic Sympathectomy (ETS)—Also see *Beating Rosacea Vascular, Ocular & Acne Forms, A Must-Have Guide to Understanding & Treating Rosacea*, Geoffrey Nase, Ph.D., Nase Publications, 2001, pages 206–208, 247
7.   *Beating Rosacea Vascular, Ocular & Acne Forms, A Must-Have Guide to Understanding & Treating Rosacea*, Geoffrey Nase, Ph.D., Nase Publications, 2001, pages 239–244
8.   ibid., page 202
9.   ibid., page 204
10. ibid., page 245–246
11. The list may include chemical peels and retinoids. Check this url >
     http://internationalrosaceafoundation.org/peels_retinoids.html
12. www.rosacea.org

A word of caution about using steroid prescription (or non-prescription) medication offered by physicians or anyone: Don't. Dr. Nase has listed 'Topical Steroids' as the fifth main trigger[14] for rosacea. Dr Nase says, "Topical steroids of any concentration should never be used to treat rosacea sufferers[15]..." The NRS lists topical steroids as one of the tripwires on their list.[16] The IRF has a page just on this subject.[17] What happens is that steroid treatment may at first relieve rosacea symptoms but later aggravates the rosacea and your rosacea gets worse. Hence, the term *steroid-induced rosacea* has developed. Ironically, uninformed physicians sometimes are the culprits triggering this rosacea and an uninformed rosacean who accepts steroid treatment can find his rosacea worse than before he began the steroid treatment. These steroid treatments are topical and you have now been warned if you are not are aware of this.

A comprehensive list of rosacea links, many to physician treatments, is on my website at this url >

http://www.rosaceans.com/html/links.html

---

13. www.rosaceainfo.com
    Note: This organization is an affiliate of the NRS. On the Rosacea Awareness Program's website it states, "The Program is funded through an educational grant by Galderma Canada, a research-based pharmaceutical company specializing in dermatology." The National Rosacea Society at the printing of this book has never publically stated the source of its funding or donations.
14. See footnote 6, page 40
15. *Beating Rosacea Vascular, Ocular & Acne Forms, A Must-Have Guide to Understanding & Treating Rosacea*, Geoffrey Nase, Ph.D., Nase Publications, 2001, pages 230–231, 286
16. *Coping with Rosacea*, National Rosacea Society, page 9
17. "'Never, never, never, ever prescribe steroids for rosacea' Dr.Kligman (Dermatology-University of Philadelphia) & Dr. Pleig (Dermatologische Klinik Und Poliklinik der Universitat Munchen, Germany) state in their 1973 book, entitled Acne & Rosacea, First edition. Likewise, their second edition in 1993 harshly criticizes dermatologists that prescribe steroids for rosacea."
    source > http://internationalrosaceafoundation.org/steroids.html

Non-Prescription Products

Based on the chapter, *Polls and Databases*, there is a significant number of rosaceans who use alternative treatment and products from non-prescription sources and many of them were mentioned there. I personally use my diet to control my rosacea along with daily sulfur soap.[1] When a pimple or stubborn spot appears on my nose or face due to cheating on my diet I use the tan disc from Rosacea LTD-III.[2] I also take grape seed extract[3] as I mention in my chapter on *Vitamins and Supplements*. My rosacea is reasonably controlled though not cured.

There are a significant number of rosacea skin care products on the market and my web site lists the ones I have heard of at this url >

http://www.rosacea-diet.com/html/non.html

and you can find both the products I use at this url >

http://www.rosacea-diet.com/html/products.html

Every rosacean has an individual condition and may use different products, so there is really no absolute treatment that works for everyone. What works for one rosacean may not work for another, as you will

---

1. Cetaphil soap is used by many rosaceans and may be more gentle to you skin
2. *Beating Rosacea Vascular, Ocular & Acne Forms, A Must-Have Guide to Understanding & Treating Rosacea*, Geoffrey Nase, Ph.D., Nase Publications, 2001, page 198 for Dr. Nase's comment on Rosacea-LTD-III
3. ibid., see page 200–201 for Dr. Nase's comment on grape seed extract which influenced me to use it.

find. That is why obtaining group information is of such great help and you should seriously consider reading the posts and information at the two groups I have formed mentioned in the chapter, *History of Posting Comments on the Internet*. Read the chapter on *Polls and Data-bases* to get an idea of what rosaceans are voting on what products they use. If you haven't got a computer you can go to any public library and use one to see what is going on. Bring this book with you to be able to enter the urls. [4]

Cosmetics

I would be remiss not to mention cosmetics for rosacea since this *always* comes up when discussing rosacea. There are a plethora of cosmetics products discussed by rosaceans in the yahoo groups formed for rosacea. Here is a partial list of a few mentioned >

Afirm	Linda Sy Skincare Products
Aromaleigh	M.D. Forte
Avéne	Mineral Secrets
Avéne	Monave
Bare Escentuals	Primacy
Belli	QVC Bare Minerals
BioElements	Reduce the Red™ Skin Care System
BioMedic	Skinceuticals
Dermalogica	Super-Skin
EstÈe Lauder Idealist Skin Refinisher	Zirh
Great Skin	
Illuminaire	
Jane Iredale	
Joey New York	
La Roche-Posay	

4. URL—Universe Resource Locator—a website address

The above cosmetics are by no means complete. There is a poll at the rosaceans group you can see what cosmetic is the most popular among rosaceans at this url >

http://groups.yahoo.com/group/rosaceans/poll

Look for the poll question > *What cosmetics are the best for rosacea?*

Sunscreens

Sunscreens also *always* come up in discussing rosacea. Sun is just about on any rosacea trigger list. So which sunscreen to use for rosacea? The choices are many but these names have come up >

BarcZone
Bull Frog
Clinique City Block Sunblock
DDF Organic Sunblock SPF 30
Dermatone UVA/UVB SPF 15
Dr. Hauschka SPF for Children
Dual Purpose
Escran Toral Phyto Aromatique
Glymed Plus
Hawaiian Tropic 45 SPF Plus UVA/UVB Broad Spectrum Sunblock
Linda Sy ZincO Cream™
Neutrogena Sunscreen for Senstive Skin
Ombrelle product line by Loreal
Peter Thomas Roth
Ti-silc
Sage Skin Care SPF 25
Z-SILK

This list is also not complete but gives you a start.[5] Go to the same url above at the rosaceans group at yahoo and look for the poll question > *What sunscreen is best for rosacea?*

---

5. *Beating Rosacea Vascular, Ocular & Acne Forms, A Must-Have Guide to Understanding & Treating Rosacea*, Geoffrey Nase, Ph.D., Nase Publications, 2001, page 196–7 for Dr. Nase's comments on sunscreens

Glycemic Index

The *Rosacea Diet* uses the carbohydrate gram as the measure to determine total carbohydrate consumption for the day. Many have known about the glycemic index and have asked me about it, but since food labels only carry the carbohydrate gram content, it is difficult to use the glycemic index as a measure when purchasing food. However, according to the Sydney University Glycemic Index Research Service (SUGiRS),

"Consumers across Australia and North America will soon know all about the glycemic index of foods via the new GI symbol on food packages. The GI symbol will appear on a range of foods that have been GI tested by an accredited testing laboratory. All of them will have been tested in 8–10 subjects using standardized methods. The actual GI will appear near the nutrition panel, along with a brief explanation."

We will look to see if this symbol appears on nutrition labels and this may be very helpful to rosaceans who desire controlling their rosacea with the *Rosacea Diet*. Future editions of the *Rosacea Diet* may cover the glycemic index, but until the GI actually appears on nutrition labels, the carbohydrate gram content is the best source of information for now. More information on this can be found at this url:

http://www.glycemicindex.com/gi_symbl.htm

Sugar Busters! uses the glycemic index and you may find out more information on how to use it which may prove useful.

About the Author

Brady Barrows (b.1950 in Boulder, Colorado) was raised in Texas by his paternal grandfather, Barney, and his step-grandmother, Beulah until age sixteen when he moved to California to live with his father, Robert Guy Barrows and step-mother, Judith Friedman Barrows. Robert & Judith at the time were television writers and Brady for the first time met his parents and brothers, Larry, David and Danny (there is also a brother Joshua and a sister Grace who came later). Brady's mother, Elizabeth Barrows, was also a television writer and married Anthony Terpiloff, also a television writer. The influence of all these screen and television writers must have had an influence on the author. Brady graduated from University High School, Los Angeles, California in 1968 and attended Santa Monica College in Santa Monica, California. He attended UCLA for a few weeks and dropped out which was what was happening in the 'tune-in, turn-on, drop-out' society of the day. If you can remember what happened during this period you really weren't there. In 1971 he moved to New Mexico and lived in the Jemez Mountains and became a hippie meeting his wife Betty whom he married. They both built a stone house on Mesa Pinabetal (near Mesa Poleo) that still stands to this day. A son, Jeremy, came along in 1973 and around this time the family became Jehovah's Witnesses. In 1994, Brady joined his wife as a full-time minister of Jehovah's Witnesses and both volunteered to do construction work for the Watchtower Bible and Tract Society, Patterson Educational Center, Patterson, New York for six months. His son Jeremy was already serving as a volunteer at the world headquarters of Jehovah's Witnesses in Brooklyn in 1994 in the production office. Brady & Betty decided to stay on the East Coast moving to Great Barrington, Massachusetts where they both have lived since. Jeremy moved to the Silicon Valley with his wife, Lillian. Brady is serving as the Secretary for the Great Barrington Congregation of Jehovah's Witnesses. Brady & Betty also work together in volunteer construction for the Massachusetts Regional Building Committee, HVAC Department, in pipe insulation on 'quickbuild kingdom halls.' Brady was diagnosed with rosacea in his thirties in New Mexico and began writing the *Rosacea Diet* in 1999. It was published by iUniverse in 2002. With the success of his first book he wrote *The Diet* for a much *larger* audience in 2003 also published by iUniverse. Both are still full-time volunteer ministers planning on moving west in 2004 after about ten years on the East Coast to a spot in the middle of the Pacific Ocean on one of the Sandwich Islands. Aloha.

Index

0-595-22800-3